FAT TO FLAT

Janet Thomson

Thorsons
An Imprint of HarperCollins*Publishers*

Thorsons
An Imprint of HarperCollins*Publishers*
77–85 Fulham Palace Road
Hammersmith, London W6 8JB
1160 Battery Street
San Francisco, California 94111–1213

Published by Thorsons 1995
10 9 8 7 6 5 4 3 2 1

A catalogue record for this book
is available from the British Library

ISBN 0 7225 3167 2

Text illustrations by Andrea Norton

Printed in Great Britain by
HarperCollinsManufacturing, Glasgow

Contents

This book is dedicated to Brian and Jean Hickford, without whom it would never have happened, and to everyone at the New Life Community Church, Lutterworth, who have been so supportive.

I would also like to thank my wonderful husband Laurie for putting up with me whilst writing it and my beautiful children Ben, Ryan and Emilie. I must also mention Sharman Thomson and thank her for her invaluable help with the recipes.

Introduction

If you are serious about wanting to lose fat, then this is definitely the book for you! In it you will find lots of information about your body – how it works and what it needs to survive – as well as how to lose fat *safely* and *effectively* – *for good*.

In this day and age, there is a huge pressure to conform to certain images of ultra skinny women or lean, muscular men. As a result of this, many 'normal' people feel inadequate and unhappy about the way they look. We have become so concerned with how we look, that we are prepared to go to almost any lengths in order to try to achieve 'The Body Beautiful' – something that, for most of us, is unachievable. Inevitably this leads to disappointment. I don't know anyone who hasn't got some part of their body which they would like to 'change', including me! Unfortunately, many people abuse their body, through months or even years of 'dieting', often without realizing it. They follow the latest 'craze' diet, taken in by false promises and expectations. Even though some of these diets result in drastic weight loss in a relatively short period of time, they can be very dangerous. As soon as you 'finish' the diet, you start to regain the weight you lost, and often lots more besides.

Regaining weight has a very negative effect on your satisfaction with your appearance, your self esteem and confidence. It usually occurs because you haven't been on a well-balanced diet, and your body wasn't getting the amount of food it needed to stay healthy whilst you were on the 'diet', or it may occur because you didn't prepare yourself for coping with 'high-risk' situations. We all need to learn how to cope with temptation, and although this aspect of weight loss is often neglected, it is *crucial* to your long-term success (*see* page 67 for more information).

In this book one of the most important things you *will* learn is how to set realistic goals. You will lose fat if you follow the guidelines set out in this book, but there will be no instant overnight change in how you look. Just as it takes a long time to become overweight, it can take a long time to lose weight safely, so that it stays off – *for good*.

So what are you expecting as you start to read this book? If you are hoping for an instant, 21-day miracle, you will be disappointed. My hope for you is that, as you read, you will learn to make changes in your life, in what you eat and in your activity levels, and that you will drastically improve your health. This has to be first and foremost. The wonderful thing about *this* book is that in addition to becoming healthier, you will also lose excess fat from your body. (That is providing you actually follow the guidelines in it, it's not enough just to read it!)

As you read, you will learn that by re-educating yourself you can become healthier *and* slimmer, at the same time. The majority of dieters feel anything from mild apprehension to dread at the thought of going on another diet. How do you feel as you are reading this? You can rest assured that this book *really is* different. I'm not trying to sell you some miracle food or potion that will solve all your problems. I have looked at weight loss from every angle, not just at what you put in your mouth! A successful weight-loss programme has to offer much more than that. I will tell you how and why you gain fat, why your body naturally changes shape as you get older, exactly what your nutritional requirements are and why many diets simply *can't* work. I will explain why exercise is so important and how to choose the best form of exercise for you, and we will also look at the psychology of dieting (why do we do it?), what you can realistically expect to achieve and, most important of all, *how* you can achieve it.

Health professionals are well aware that in order

to achieve long-term weight loss, long-term changes in behaviour must take place. This means changing eating habits, as well as including some kind of exercise regime, however gentle. As a profession we are all united on this issue – there is no debate. We know it is the truth. In spite of this some unscrupulous companies, more interested in their bank balance than in our health, spend millions of pounds each year trying to convince us that the next 'Quick Fix' is just around the corner, that their latest 'discovery' really is *the* one which will rid us of those unwanted inches in record time – *false*.

This kind of marketing is very cruel.

The truth is, *none* of the 'quick-fix' diets, including meal-replacement drinks and many other pills and potions, will work in the long term (*see* Chapter 2 to find out why). As soon as you return to your original way of eating, you are repeating the process which made you overweight in the first place. In the meantime, your body has been messed about so much that it is convinced it is going to be 'starved', so it learns to store fat more efficiently in order to conserve fuel.

Consumers are very vulnerable to advertisements and clever marketing strategies, and there is a desperate need to educate people so that they are not taken in by false claims.

I have written this book in order to dispel the myths. It is probably the most important book you will ever read, and I would encourage you to read all of it, from cover to cover. You will also find it very valuable to 'dip into' from time to time, to remind yourself about certain things.

I wish you success. My goal is to help you achieve your goal, whatever that may be. Whether you want to lose four stones, or three pounds, this book will help you to achieve it, and also to become fitter, healthier and to get more out of life. That has to be good!

Chapter 1

Nutrition – The Bare Necessities

*The Nutrients You Need
and How to Get Them*

How much do you really know about nutrition? My guess is that you probably already know that what you eat isn't ideal. Does this sound familiar?

My diet is horrendous, I just don't have the time to eat properly. I often skip breakfast, it's too much of a rush. I have a light lunch, sometimes a bag of crisps and a sandwich, or just a piece of fruit. I have several cups of tea or coffee during the day, sometimes with a biscuit, and my largest meal in the evening, which leaves me feeling full up and bloated. I know I should make more of an effort, but I just can't.

How often have you felt a sense of frustration, or even failure, because you know you're not doing the best for your body? It's no wonder we turn to the quick-fix diets that promise magical results in short periods of time, only to find out that they don't work and that we often end up worse than before we started.

In this chapter I will give you an outline of the basic food groups: what they are and why we need them; how much we need to stay healthy; and how the energy nutrients are broken down to provide us with fuel. I will also give you tips to help you put it all in to practice.

Why do we need nutritious food? The answer is quite simple – to provide our body with everything it needs to be able to function well, to give us the energy we need to go about daily life and to help prevent illness. It's not enough just to fill our bodies with bulk to get rid of hunger pangs, we need a balance of nutrients in order to achieve optimum health.

I believe the key to changing eating (and exercise) habits is learning to understand the body's needs. How often do we accept a new pill or powder just because it *says* it's full of nourishment? If we can understand what the body needs, how much of it, and *why*, it becomes much easier to see where we're going wrong and to do something about it.

So what is a 'diet'? Going on a 'diet' doesn't necessarily mean you are reducing the amount you eat in order to lose weight. Everyone is on a diet; it simply means what you eat. You shouldn't think of the recommendations in this book as something you should do, or 'go on', but, as I explained in the Introduction, as reasons and ways to change – *permanently*. After all, if you can 'go on' a diet, then you can also 'come off' it, and then you are back to square one.

Let's find out how much you do know about nutrition. With all the clever marketing that major food companies produce, it *is* difficult to tell fact from fiction. Test your knowledge with these questions and see how you do:

1. Only fat, carbohydrate and protein give us energy.   true/false
2. Protein can be stored as fat.   true/false
3. Alcohol can be used to provide muscular energy.   true/false
4. Carbohydrate provides us with twice as many calories as fat per gram.   true/false
5. You have to eat meat to get adequate supplies of protein.   true/false
6. Protein is essential for hormone production.   true/false
7. There are approximately 21 essential amino acids (proteins).   true/false
8. A deficiency of even one of these amino acids can impair growth.   true/false
9. Potatoes contain protein.   true/false
10. A high-protein diet is potentially very dangerous.   true/false
11. Meat is a good source of zinc and vitamin B_{12}.   true/false

12. Fat vitamins are soluble in water.   true/false
13. Essential fatty acids (EFAs) reduce your risk of heart disease.   true/false
14. Margarines containing hydrogenated fats are bad for you; butter only contains natural ingredients and so is a better choice from a health point of view.   true/false
15. Cholesterol is a fatty substance found in animal fat.   true/false
16. The body can produce cholesterol if you don't take it in through food.   true/false
17. Carbohydrate should make up the largest portion of our diet.   true/false
18. In order to burn fat you must eat carbohydrate.   true/false
19. Dietary fibre cannot be broken down by the body.   true/false
20. A diet too high in fibre takes out essential vitamins and minerals.   true/false
21. Minerals are essential for blood clotting.   true/false
22. Vitamins can be manufactured by the body.   true/false

Here are the answers, have a look and see how you did. The correct answer is shown in italics.

1. Only fat, carbohydrate and protein give us energy. *true*/false
2. Protein can be stored as fat. *true*/false
3. Alcohol can be used to provide muscular energy. true/*false*
4. Carbohydrate provides us with twice as many calories as fat per gram. true/*false*
5. You have to eat meat to get adequate supplies of protein. true/*false*
6. Protein is essential for hormone production. *true*/false
7. There are approximately 21 essential amino acids (proteins). *true*/false
8. A deficiency of even one of these amino acids can impair growth. *true*/false
9. Potatoes contain protein. *true*/false
10. A high-protein diet is potentially very dangerous. *true*/false
11. Meat is a good source of zinc and vitamin B_{12}. *true*/false
12. Fat vitamins are soluble in water. true/*false*
13. Essential fatty acids (EFAs) reduce your risk of heart disease. *true*/false
14. Margarines containing hydrogenated fats are bad for you; butter only contains natural

ingredients and so is a better choice from a health
point of view   *true*/false

15. Cholesterol is a fatty substance found in
    animal fat.   *true*/false

16. The body can produce cholesterol if you don't
    take it in through food.   *true*/false

17. Carbohydrate should make up the largest
    portion of our diet.   *true*/false

18. In order to burn fat you must eat carbohydrate.
                                                     true/false

19. Dietary fibre cannot be broken down by the
    body.   *true*/false

20. A diet too high in fibre takes out essential
    vitamins and minerals.   *true*/false

21. Minerals are essential for blood clotting.
                                                     true/false

22. Vitamins can be manufactured by the body.
                                                     true/*false*

How did you do? If you got some of them wrong, you
will learn a lot of valuable information in this chapter
that will help you to achieve your goal.

THE ESSENTIAL NUTRIENTS

The foods or nutrients we eat can be broken down
into six groups:

- carbohydrates
- fat
- protein
- vitamins
- minerals
- water

The first three are our **energy nutrients**; in other words, they contain the fuel our bodies need to be able to function effectively. We burn calories, not only when we exercise but all the time, in order for our bodies to function and stay healthy. A 'calorie' is simply a way of measuring the amount of energy we are using. One calorie represents the amount of heat energy it takes to raise the temperature of 1 gram of water by 1°C. A 'kilocalorie' represents 1000 calories. This is often written as Calorie (capital C), which means the same thing. All the calories from food come from carbohydrate, fat and protein, and this is why they are called the energy nutrients.

CARBOHYDRATES

Carbohydrates come essentially from plants, in other words, they have grown organically. They can be classified as foods which 'have not been born'. For example, pasta, rice, potatoes, vegetables and breads are all carbohydrates, and none of them have a mother. They are of organic origin. Plants capture the energy in sunlight and use it to produce glucose. When we eat plants, we are eating valuable sources of glucose which our bodies can then break down and use as energy.

Carbohydrates can be classified into two groups: simple sugars and complex carbohydrates. On their own, **simple sugars** – such as glucose, fructose, lactose and sucrose – are 'empty' calories. They have no significant nutritional value whatsoever, they just make things taste sweet. Unfortunately, sugar is added to many foods during processing, you only need to look at the food labels on everyday items such as baked beans to find examples. More obvious food sources include:

- sweets
- sugars
- honey

Complex carbohydrates are organic foods which also contain stores of starch. They are more complex in their make up, which consists of a combination of vitamins, minerals and fibre. Unlike simple sugars, they have a very high nutritional value and should make up the largest proportion of our diet. Good sources include:

- fruit
- vegetables
- grains

Many people have misconceptions about the amount of carbohydrate they should eat if they are on a weight-reducing diet. For example, bread, potatoes and pasta are on the 'forbidden' list of many diet sheets. *Wrong*! This is *bad* advice! Carbohydrates are not fattening, *fat* is fattening! It is the fat (butter etc.) which you put on the bread and potatoes that makes them fattening and *not* the carbohydrates themselves. However, if the total number of calories you consume in one day is higher than the number you burn, then you will gain weight as your body stores the excess as fat.

Recent research suggests that a diet which is high in carbohydrate and low in fat reduces the risk of developing some forms of cancer. This is because carbohydrates contain valuable nutrients which act as antioxidants. These antioxidants can deactivate harmful chemicals in the body, particularly if the carbohydrates are eaten fresh and raw. These harmful chemicals are known as 'free radicals', which attack and injure vital cell structures. If you eat plenty of raw vegetables such as:

- carrots
- spinach

- watercress
- asparagus
- broccoli
- green peppers
- Brussels sprouts
- cauliflower
- red cabbage

fruit, such as:

- peaches
- apricots
- oranges
- bananas
- apples
- strawberries

and some nuts and whole-grains, such as wheat, you will be getting an excellent supply of natural anti-oxidants. These valuable antioxidants can help protect the body against many degenerative diseases, such as heart disease.

Remember: carbohydrates are a *good* source of fuel. They also provide valuable vitamins and minerals. If they are eaten in moderation, they will not make you fat. However, don't forget, too much of anything will be converted to and stored as body fat.

FAT

Fat is an excellent source of energy and performs many essential functions within the body. Certain vitamins can only be obtained from fat, and these are crucial for maintaining the nutritional balance we need. Fat holds your internal organs in place, makes up a large percentage of your brain, and helps to connect your skin to your framework. It is, therefore, certainly *not* advisable to go on a fat-free diet.

You may have heard the term **essential fatty acids (EFAs)**. This simply means fats that are essential for the body to maintain optimum health. Our body cannot manufacture these types of fat, so we must include them in our diet. The two essential fatty acids are called Omega 3 or Alpha linolenic, which is found in oily fish, and Omega 6 or cis linoleic, which is found in vegetable oils. Another fatty acid called arachidonic acid is semi-essential, as our body can make it, providing it has an adequate supply of other nutrients.

Essential fatty acids are vital for the health of your heart and circulation systems, as well as many other bodily functions. Not getting enough EFAs can lead to a deterioration in health and ultimately in death (deficiency symptoms are listed below). EFAs are found in safflower, sunflower, corn, sesame, pumpkin and linseed oils. Other good food sources include green vegetables, soya, fish (e.g. salmon, mackerel, rainbow trout and sardines), and fish oils. Although all whole, fresh, unprocessed foods contain some EFAs, these EFAs go through many changes in the body, as the body has to break down and refine them into substances it can use. Many of us take in enough EFAs through the diet but, unfortunately, we also take in other foods which block the breakdown of the EFAs and prevent them from doing their valuable work. These foods include saturated fat, cholesterol, large amounts of alcohol and high levels of sugar. We should, therefore, not only think about how much fat we need, but also look at the quality of the fat we are taking in. If you consider that every single cell in your body contains fat to support its membrane, you can see why the right quality is so important. If we don't take in enough of the good quality fats we can't use them to make our cells. Would you really like to be made from second-class materials?

If you're not getting enough EFAs, symptoms can include:

- eczema or dry skin
- hair loss
- liver/kidney degeneration
- excessive water loss
- susceptibility to infections
- failure to heal
- inflammatory conditions such as arthritis

- heart and circulatory problems
- deterioration of vision
- muscle nerve-impulse breakdown
- loss of motor skills – the ability to control muscular actions

And so the list goes on. With many other major and minor conditions now being linked to a lack of EFAs, it is *vital* that we take in sufficient quantities through our diet, and also avoid foods that stop our body from utilizing these precious nutrients.

Having established the importance of the EFAs, it is worth considering that most of us still eat far more dietary fat than we need and eat fat of poor quality, in other words, too much of the bad stuff and not enough of the good stuff! We store this surplus as fat on our body. A high intake of the wrong kinds of fat drastically increases the likelihood of heart disease, heart attacks and many other serious illness.

The fat we eat is broken down into fatty acids, which will do one of two things: either it will be used to produce energy, or it will be placed into storage, in the fat cells. This stored fat is called *adipose tissue*. It is also sometimes called *cellulite*. The only way that fat comes out of fat cells is when it is to be burnt as fuel. Fat will not be broken down by any cream or potion; it is a fuel and any excess has to be burnt.

The fat cell is constantly active, with fat going in

and coming out all the time. If you maintain a balance between what you burn and what you consume you won't get fatter. If the balance is tipped the wrong way, however, and you eat more than you burn, the fat cells will increase in size (*see* page 75 for facts about fat).

Fat is either saturated (i.e. solid at room temperature) or unsaturated (i.e. liquid at room temperature). Most **saturated fats** are of animal origin (exceptions include palm oil and coconut oil), and contain high levels of cholesterol, which is another fatty substance present in animal fat. Cholesterol can clog up arteries and restrict blood flow if consumed in excess.

Cholesterol can be divided up into 'good' cholesterol (HDL) or 'bad' cholesterol (LDL). It is the ratio between the two that is important. LDL carries cholesterol around the body and deposits excess amounts in the blood vessels. HDL mops up this excess and carries it back to the liver, where it can be broken down and excreted by the body (fibre helps this process). If the level of LDL is much higher than the level of HDL, then more and more cholesterol gets deposited in the blood vessels, which can ultimately lead to a blockage. Although every cell in the body has a need for cholesterol, the body is able to manufacture all that we need providing we are eating a nutritionally balanced diet.

It is saturated fat that has been associated with

heart disease. One way of restricting your intake of both saturated fat and cholesterol is to reduce the amount of meat you eat, and to always choose lean cuts. Despite popular belief, beef is not exceptionally high in cholesterol and, in this respect, can be compared equally with chicken or fish. However, the total saturated fat content of beef is relatively high, and it should therefore be eaten in moderation.

Unsaturated fats are considered to be more 'healthy'. In fact, one particular unsaturated fat, extra virgin olive oil, seems to be health-protective. A sprinkling of this oil on a salad or when cooking a stir fry is a good way of getting the essential vitamins provided by fat without the associated problems of saturated fats.

Fish is another good source of high-quality fat, in particular oily fish such as salmon, mackerel, tuna and sardines. The oils found in these fish can help prevent heart disease, as they block many harmful reactions which can cause blood to overclot. The way you prepare your fish is also very important; don't fry it in butter or cover it in a creamy sauce! If you don't like fish, you may have been tempted by the range of fish oil capsules currently on the market. Some of the higher quality brands, available in good health-food shops, are well worth taking. Always read the label and ask for advice before you buy – assistants in health-food shops are usually quite knowledgeable with regard to the best kind of supplements, so take their advice. When you actually look at the amount of nutrients you are getting for your money, the more expensive brands often work out cheaper in the long run, as more of the nutrients can be absorbed by the body than in some of the cheaper alternatives.

It is worth remembering that fat is often hidden behind other names when used in menus and recipes. For example, cream is essentially fat, but somehow 'Fat of Chicken Soup' or an 'Ice Fat' doesn't sound quite so appetizing does it? In reality, however, that is exactly what you would be eating. Just ask yourself, 'Do I want to wear this chocolate bar more than I want to eat it?'

Remember: some fat is essential, so select high-quality oils and keep to a minimum the amount of saturated fat you eat. The menus in this book have been carefully planned to give you the right balance of EFAs, whilst minimizing the amount of saturated fat.

PROTEIN

Proteins are often referred to as the 'building blocks' of the body. This is because our muscles are made up of tiny strands of protein called amino acids, which give the body its basic shape and support. As we are constantly breaking down these strands, they have to be continually replaced. Protein's other vital roles include: maintaining healthy skin, hair and nails; the production of hormones; sexual development; and sustaining healthy levels of red blood cells (which carry oxygen around the body). Although it is the second most plentiful substance in the body – after water – of all three energy nutrients, it is also the one we need least of. As with *fat*, it's the quality of the protein we eat that determines our health. Providing we are eating enough calories per day to satisfy our individual requirements, we will usually be taking in more than we actually need – so don't worry about the quantity.

Protein is broken down in the body into many different **amino acids**. The body is able to manufacture some of these itself, but there are eight essential amino acids which cannot be manufactured. A deficiency of even one of these eight can lead to problems with the production of protein structures.

Foods which are rich in protein do not always contain all the essential amino acids. If the food does contain all eight it is termed *complete*, and foods that are low in one or more termed *incomplete*. Most meats and dairy products are complete protein foods, whilst most vegetables and fruits are incomplete. Ideally we should eat a mixture of animal and vegetable sources to ensure that we are getting the full complement. It is possible to get all the required amino acids from fruit and vegetables, but foods must be carefully selected. Vegetarians should take care to include beans, lentils and pulses in at least two of their meals each day. They should also combine incomplete proteins, such as grains (i.e. cereals, pasta and breads), with milk or milk products (such as cheese or yogurt). Grains can be combined with beans and legumes to achieve the same effect, and seeds can also be a good source of protein if combined with legumes. The proteins obtainable from vegetable sources are not as easily absorbed as those from meat sources. Vitamin C can aid this process, so vegetarians should always eat or drink foods rich in this vitamin with their meal, for example, an orange or a glass of orange juice.

Animal Sources of Protein
- meat
- meat products (pâté, offal)
- fish
- fish products (paste etc.)
- shellfish
- cheese (although watch the fat content)
- yogurt
- eggs
- milk

Vegetable Sources of Protein
- beans
- lentils

- peas (including chick peas)
- butter beans
- textured vegetable protein – TVP (often used as a filler in commercial products)
- Quorn (a meat alternative)
- nuts and nut products
- bread
- potatoes
- cereals
- rice
- pasta (preferably whole-wheat)

The body takes what protein it needs from these foods and breaks it down into amino acids which can then be used by the body – but it is unable to store the rest as protein. (If you think about it, we don't have spare muscles tucked away do we?) Any protein left over is stored as fat, along with everything else we take in excess (for information about the dangers of high-protein diets, *see* page 42).

The Energy Nutrients – Picking the Right Combinations

A combination of all three energy nutrients is essential to maintain optimum health and to provide us with all the energy we need for everyday life. What we need most of is *carbohydrate*, which should make up approximately 60–65 per cent of our diet; next in line is *fat*, which should make up 25–30 per cent maximum; and lastly, protein, which should make up the remaining percentage.

If you think of your favourite meal (roast beef, Yorkshire pudding, roast potatoes and vegetables, or lamb chops with chips and peas, for example), you probably list the protein element first and foremost and plan your meal around that. When you look at your plate, foods from the carbohydrate group should take up most of the room – vegetables and rice, for example. The smallest portion should be from the high-protein foods, such as meat and fish. If this is what you see, then it is likely that you are achieving the correct balance between carbohydrate, fat and protein – well done! If most of the space on your plate is taken up by the meat or fish, you definitely need to make some changes. People rarely achieve the correct balance, however, and the protein often makes up at least half of the meal. Because many protein sources, such as meat and cheese, are high in fat (often saturated), the balance is tipped the wrong way and the majority of the meal is then made up of fat calories. This not only increases the size of your fat cells, but also increases your risk of suffering from heart disease or attack.

Food and Fibre
Dietary fibre comes from plant foods and is the only

component of food that cannot be broken down by the gut. This means that it comes out the same as it goes in. Fibre keeps the gut mobile, which is very important. Some research has indicated that this may be cancer-protective. By eating more fibre you can also decrease your cholesterol level, which helps to reduce the risk of heart disease. Good sources of fibre include:

- fruit
- vegetables
- legumes
- whole grains

Processed food loses much of its fibre content, often because the skin is removed from fruit and whole-wheat flour milled into white flour. The brown varieties of bread and rice generally contain more fibre than their white counterparts.

If you are eating a wide variety of carbohydrate foods you will automatically be getting enough fibre. Diets which are too high in fibre can be harmful, as food passes through the gut before the digestive system has had time to extract all the nutrients. High-fibre diets require an increase in the amount of water consumed, as water will be absorbed into the fibre. If you do eat lots of fibre and don't drink enough water, you may develop extreme stomach cramps.

VITAMINS

Vitamins are manufactured by plants, including fruits, vegetables and other foods from the carbo-hydrate group. The word 'vitamin' means 'vital' and vitamins are indeed essential for life. They play an important role in the formation of red blood cells, bone building and many other functions of the body.

There are two different types of vitamin: fat soluble and water soluble. *Fat-soluble* vitamins – A, D, E and K – are absorbed along with fat. The body usually has a plentiful store of these vitamins and an excess can lead to the body becoming poisoned by them. *Water-soluble* vitamins – B complex and C – are more easily excreted by the body, via urine. Taking extreme quantities, however, can lead to dangerous and unpleasant side effects, such as permanent damage to the liver.

Vitamin supplementation is big business these days. Powerful marketing strategies are used to sell us various combinations of pills and capsules, and many people have become convinced that in order to stay healthy they must supplement their food intake. In some cases supplements are used instead of meals. I recently asked a friend of mine, who regularly complains of a lack of energy, what he'd had for breakfast. 'I've had a multi-vitamin tablet and I'm full up,' he replied! There is a great danger here. Vitamin supplements can be very beneficial in cases of deficiency, as prescribed by a dietician or nutritionist. When sold over the counter, however, they can be misused and can cause more problems than they solve.

In an ideal world there would be a plentiful supply of vitamins in the foods we eat. If you eat a wide variety of foods you *should* automatically get all the nutrients you require. Much of our food is over-processed, however, and so has lost a lot of its nutritional value before it reaches our saucepan. It then loses even more value during the cooking process, which means that there is very little left by the time we actually eat it. To minimize this loss, it's well worth buying organically grown produce wherever possible. Although it is more expensive, you do get a lot more real food for your money.

If you decide that you do need to supplement, I recommend that you take advice from a qualified nutritionist or dietician before you buy. The way in which the body absorbs vitamins is very finely tuned; it requires a certain amount of each one. If one particular vitamin is taken in excess, the whole balance may be disrupted and the body's ability to absorb other vitamins impaired. Vegetarians are one group who do need to supplement, as they do not get the valuable B_{12} vitamin which has many vital functions in the body. A deficiency of B_{12} can lead to anaemia, so all vegetarians should take a multivitamin that includes B$_{12}$ (the recommended amount per day is a minimum of 1.5mcg).

At the end of the day, if there is a deficiency in your diet, that should be the first thing you look into rather than a pill bottle. It is likely that you are not eating something you should be. With the correct advice this can be easily rectified. If you are sure that you are getting a well-balanced diet and still have symptoms of deficiency – take advice.

MINERALS

Minerals are present in all living cells. They perform many important functions in the human body. Bones and teeth, for example, are made from living tissue combined with various minerals. Minerals are also essential for nerve transmission and many other metabolic functions. Some minerals are required in large amounts, such as calcium and phosphorus; others in smaller quantities, such as iron and zinc. As with vitamins, eating a varied diet should ensure that you get all the minerals you need. This will depend, however, on the quality of the foods you eat, and if you're not sure, take qualified advice.

One way of ensuring that you extract all the vitamins and minerals from your food is to avoid tea and coffee, particularly at meal times. Substances in these drinks can drastically reduce the body's ability to absorb nourishment, sometimes by as much as 50 per cent. Try to avoid them for at least half an hour before and after your meal, or better still, don't have them at all. I have recently changed from tea to a caffeine-free instant drink, made from roasted barley rye and chicory – it's delicious and I don't miss tea one bit.

GOOD FOODS AND BAD FOODS

How do you tell the difference between a 'good' food and a 'bad' one? The answer is that there are no bad foods. I believe in everything in moderation. One chocolate biscuit isn't going to do you any harm at all, it's the rest of the packet that really does the damage! If you can eat one and be satisfied, great, lucky you! Most of us 'mere mortals' cannot resist the temptation and just *have to* delve deeper into the packet.

There are, of course, healthy foods and non-healthy foods and, if you educate your stomach and palate and get used to low-fat foods, even chocolate loses its appeal – I promise! Speaking as someone who used to devour two or three chocolate bars a day, I always considered myself lucky that I rarely gained weight; that is, until I got to 30, when, it seems, all your bad habits finally catch up with you! Suddenly I had to start watching what I ate and chocolate was the first thing to go. It took me about four weeks to stop wanting a chocolate-fix, but now I don't even miss it. I have strayed a couple of times, only to find that I still can't have just one chocolate on its own. So for me the only way to do it is to not have any at all. As for other so-called bad foods, like fish and chips, if you only have them once in a while, you won't suddenly put inches on your thighs after just one meal. If you develop a taste for them, however, and have them regularly, the inches will start to pile on.

NUTRITION – CHANGE WITHOUT PAIN

In order to make the necessary changes in your diet you have to change the way you shop. After all, with the best intentions in the world, you can only cook the foods you buy. One factor that puts a lot of people off dieting is the thought of buying and preparing special foods and recipes. With this plan, however, you can eat a lot of the foods you are eating already; you simply change the quantities and the way in which the food is prepared.

Don't expect to get everything right overnight. If you've got to retrain your shopping habits and your palate, give yourself time to adapt and experiment. If you force yourself to eat food you don't enjoy because it's 'good for you', you won't stick to it. Remember, this *isn't* a diet that you go on then come off: these are lifestyle changes that really will improve the quality of your life *forever*. Food is one of the pleasures of life, and one man's pleasure is another man's poison. So if you don't see menus which you like in this book, try to adapt the foods which you already eat. *Anyone can do it.*

You could put all of your family on a highly nutritious low-fat diet and they wouldn't even notice the difference.

TIPS FOR SUCCESS

1. Fill your Shopping Trolley with Carbohydrates

Buy More	*Buy Less*
Cereals (check sugar content)	Meat
Bread	Dairy produce
Pasta (egg-free & whole-wheat)	Eggs (two per week)
Rice	Nuts (vegetarians only)
Vegetables (all colours and textures)	Sugar
Fruit (all colours and textures)	
Potatoes (don't fry them or cover them in butter)	
Oily fish	

I used to curse the design of supermarkets. It seemed so illogical! Everything always ended up balanced onto and squashed into the trolley. Most supermarkets, however, are in fact perfectly designed for low-fat, healthy shopping. The first aisle is where the vegetables are and we should start filling the trolley right there. Buy anything that looks good, especially organic produce if possible. Experiment with vegetables that you haven't tried before. Instead of having one vegetable on your plate with your meat and potatoes, have less meat and two or three different vegetables – it's cheaper too!

The second aisle is usually where you will find rice and pasta, which is great – more carbohydrate. Try different varieties, there's a wide range to choose from. With pasta and rice, however, do try and stick to the unrefined egg-free, whole-wheat varieties wherever possible.

Aisle number three is home to the cereals. By the time we finish this aisle the trolley should be two-thirds full, leaving only space for a small amount of meat. If you usually buy 1lb/500g of mince for a spaghetti bolognese, buy half, plus an extra tin of tomatoes, more mushrooms, onions, peppers and any other vegetables you like. You'll find that you can make exactly the same quantity and no one will notice the difference. Now there should be just enough room for domestic items and no room at all for chocolate biscuits!

2. Always Have Breakfast

Breakfast really is the most important meal of the day. Of all the possible mistakes you could make when planning your meals, missing breakfast is probably the worst. I am frequently being told, 'I don't have time,' or 'I'm not hungry.' A recent comment was 'I don't like breakfast foods.' Quite honestly, these are all feeble excuses, so let's examine them one at a time.

A. *Lack of time.* Eating breakfast doesn't necessarily have to be the first thing you do every morning. If you have to leave early for work, take breakfast with you – a yogurt, fruit, or some dried cereal in a plastic container, for example. Eat it mid-morning or when it is convenient. If you rise at six, you should eat it before ten, if possible. The same applies if you have to get children to school – have it after nine o'clock, when you get back. There are other things we have to do in the morning because our body needs to, whether we like it or not! How many of us would cancel the trip to the toilet to gain a few extra minutes to get ready? It's just as well that we don't have the choice – our bodily functions take over! Breakfast is also a necessary function.

B. *Not being hungry*. People who don't eat breakfast and have little or no lunch usually work up a hefty appetite by the evening, and consume more calories throughout the evening, often devouring biscuits and other high-calorie foods. These eating patterns can reduce the morning appetite, so breakfast is missed again, and the cycle repeats itself. People think that if they don't eat all day, they can then eat as much as they like in the evening. Wrong! This is the time when the body burns fewer calories because we are less active, so we are more likely to store it as fat.

C. *Disliking breakfast foods*. There are no *set* breakfast foods. Although we traditionally eat cereals and toast, there's no law that says we have to. I had this discussion one day during a talk I was giving on nutrition. One particular lady was adamant that she couldn't have breakfast because she didn't like it. I asked her to think of a favourite, easily prepared lunch and she came up with beans on toast. 'Why not have that for breakfast? It sounds ideal, a low-fat, carbohydrate mixture. What's the problem?' I asked. 'You just don't have beans on toast for breakfast,' she said. Wrong! You can have whatever you like, whenever you like it. I have often finished up the stew from the previous night with a slice of bread for breakfast – when I open the fridge I just can't resist the smell! If my work load is particularly heavy and the children are waking me up at night, I often suffer from mouth ulcers, which make eating very painful. When this happens, I have a large bowl of rice pudding for breakfast, made with skimmed milk.

Don't get stuck in the breakfast rut: vary the foods you have so that you enjoy breakfast as much as your evening meal. When you wake up, think of something low-fat that you'd like to eat, and eat it!

People who do skip breakfast are likely to suffer from a lack of energy throughout the morning, until they have something to eat. This will lead to reduced performance and often irritability or headaches. Whether it's at home doing the housework, or working in the office, productivity levels will be low. The time you saved by not having breakfast is then lost tenfold because your body cannot function at its best. Breakfast kick-starts the metabolism for the day and is a *must*, whether you are trying to lose weight or not.

3. Plan your Meals

If you have little or no breakfast, you are more likely to reach for that mid-morning snack, a packet of crisps or coffee and biscuits. A small lunch means hunger by the evening, and if you are too hungry, you'll eat the first thing you can lay your hands on – healthy or not. This is the time when the temptation to go down to the chip shop sets in and this can be hard to resist.

One of the best gifts I ever received was a slow cooker. When I'm working it takes just five minutes in the morning – or the night before – to put some vegetables and meat into the pot with some water and a few spices. By the time I come home, the smell oozing from the kitchen is wonderful. In the time that it takes to boil some rice or potatoes I have a satisfying, healthy dinner. I have also made bolognese sauce, stews and curries in this way, and the extra cooking time always adds to the flavour and makes the meat really tender.

For lunch I often raid the fridge for cold vegetables, which I mix together with some low-fat mayonnaise and cold rice. I take this in a plastic container to eat at work when I'm hungry. This removes the temptation to buy sandwiches and other goodies from the bakery.

4. Satisfy Yourself at Each Meal Time
This doesn't mean eat as much as you can, it means eat until you are reasonably full. Don't rush your food. The brain doesn't receive the message from the stomach that it's full for about 20 minutes, so wait a

while after you've eaten a meal. If you think you are still hungry after 20 minutes and the hunger pangs are still there, have a little more – if not, don't. It's always a good idea to have a starter with your main meal, as your brain then starts to receive messages of fullness from the stomach as you are beginning your main course. Choose low-fat starters that take a while to eat, such as soup and bread, or croutons with low-fat dips. Hopefully this will leave little or no room for that fattening dessert!

EATING OUT

How often have you started a diet with the best intentions, gone out for a meal a few days later and eaten all the foods you know you shouldn't, felt like you'd blown the diet completely and then given up? Sounds familiar? I hear this all the time from people who think that one lapse means that everything they've achieved over the past few days or weeks has gone out the window. Whilst I don't recommend lots of eating out when you are trying to lose weight, the last thing I want is for you to feel like you *can't* go out. After all, that's the one thing that will make you crave a restaurant meal more than anything else.

There are, however, a few guidelines which you should observe. Firstly, go to a restaurant you know, where the chef doesn't mind making alterations to some of the dishes. I always ask for a low-fat sauce and no butter, for example. If you are going somewhere for the first time, make the reservation yourself and ask then if the chef can prepare you something low-fat in advance, including dessert. This is much better than asking when you get there and he doesn't have time.

Indian restaurants are probably the worst if you are trying to lose weight. Even so, it is possible to choose something low in fat and high in taste. Stick to tandoori dishes, particularly tandoori fish or chicken. Tikka dishes are also fine. Some sauces are yogurt-based rather than cream-based, and these are OK providing the meat isn't too fatty. You will need to ask for details, as each restaurant will have it's own variety of the same dish. Watch out for the vegetable side dishes, which are often dripping in oil – ask them to cook you one with no oil. Vegetable curry can also be a good choice, with some plain boiled rice. If you have naan bread, make sure you ask them not to put butter on it.

The dishes to avoid completely are the ones that contain creamy sauces, such as a korma, and also the fried rice. They are literally loaded with fat calories – you may well carry the memory of your evening out for a very long time if you have one of these! For dessert have a sorbet – most Indian restaurants have a selection of different flavours. Not only are sorbets fat-free, but they will also clear and refresh your mouth.

Chinese restaurants are probably second on the hit list, as they use large amounts of oil. I ask what type of oil they use and have always been told vegetable oil – because it's cheap and they use so much. You only have to look at an empty plate after you've eaten a Chinese meal to see the grease that's been left behind – you could write your name in it!

If you go to a Chinese restaurant that you know cooks the food to order, ask them to cook yours with little or no fat. If they agree to do this – and most will – you can enjoy a really nice meal without worrying too much. Chinese restaurants often offer a steamed fish, and may also steam you some vegetables to go with it. This would be ideal with boiled rice. Again, you could ask for this in advance when you make your reservation. Dishes to avoid are anything containing red meat or duck and, of course, that fried rice. Prawn crackers are like sponges that soak up the fat and should also always be avoided. For dessert, as with Indian restaurants, stick to a sorbet – definitely no toffee bananas! And finally, you may find a lot of Chinese food very salty, which will probably make you drink more. Don't forget that too much wine or beer will also contribute to the total amount of calories you consume during the meal.

Italian restaurants usually offer both extremes. On

the one hand you'll probably find very rich foods in creamy sauces with lots of red meat, and at the other end of the scale you can normally get a vegetable bolognese sauce with some pasta and a salad (watch out for the salad dressing!) This second meal would be fine, or equally a small pizza, which, if you request it, can be cooked with little or no cheese. Watch out too for olives – they are over 90 per cent fat! Although they are a very good source of quality fat, one or two should be sufficient – if you have them all over your salad or pizza you will definitely be getting more than you need in one meal. You'll often find a larger selection of desserts than with the Indian or Chinese restaurants, and should be able to get a delicious fresh fruit salad (you could always take a small pot of fromage frais to pour over it if they don't have any!)

Fast-food restaurants are a disaster if you are trying to lose weight and should therefore be avoided. Exceptions to this are certain pizza restaurants who now do a vegetable bolognese sauce to go with pasta and a salad from the salad bar (the dressings, however, are not low in fat). They also do delicious fat-free yogurt for dessert, so if I want to take the children out for a meal, this is usually where we go.

If you do go to a burger restaurant ask them which fat they use. I have been told that one of the larger chains uses animal fat (saturated) to deep fry the chips – so if you find out which one it is, go to another one instead! Better still, don't go to any. Don't be taken in by claims that the burgers come from 100 per cent beef; remember, cows contain lots of unpleasant fatty bits that we definitely don't need to eat. The 100 per cent beef promise doesn't mean you only get the good bits, it could be 100 per cent of the rubbish no one else wants!

Chapter 2

Busting the Body Myths

Diets Demystified and the Facts of Fat

There is so much misinformation about how to lose weight, that it's not surprising people don't know which way to turn when a new 'product' comes out. My heart sinks whenever I hear of new fads and gimmicks that are on the market, and I grieve for all the people taken in by false promises and clever marketing. I believe it is emotional blackmail: 'Try this pill/potion/drink and, hey presto, no more fat.'

Have you been taken in by the quick-fix products? If you have had a weight problem for some time, then I'd be surprised if you hadn't. After all, faced with the choice of taking a pill or going on a diet to lose weight, don't we always want to take the easy option? Of course we do, it's human nature. Unfortunately, as I have already mentioned, none of these products actually work. They may even harm you and promote weight gain, which would of course make you a perfect customer for the next product to come along.

I was speaking to a friend recently who is in her mid-30s and suffers from acne and spots (at least she thinks she does, I hadn't noticed before!) She said, 'Janet, I never learn. I have tried every potion and lotion on the market, and yet each time a new one comes out I think this is the one that's going to do it – but it never does.' Does this sound familiar? Is this how you feel about every 'miracle diet' that comes along? Let's look at a few of the myths that surround the diet industry. Here are some of the most common misconceptions.

Potatoes and pasta make you fat.
False. Both of these foods are carbohydrates and can make up a valuable portion of our diet – it's what you put on them that normally causes the problem. A jacket potato smothered in butter will certainly be high in fat. If it is filled with raw vegetables in a low-fat dressing, however, it can make a nutritious low-fat meal or snack. Pasta, too, contains very little fat itself (providing you buy the durum-wheat variety and not one that contains egg). A pasta salad provides lots of nutrients for a tasty meal. Both potatoes and pasta are quite slow to release carbohydrate – this means that they release glucose into our blood gradually over a period of time, giving us a constant supply of energy. As a result of this, you won't feel full up one minute and hungry an hour later. Of course, too much of

anything will cause you to gain weight, including carbohydrate. If the total amount of calories you consume is greater than the total amount you burn, the excess will be stored – as fat.

If I diet I will only lose fat from one part of my body – so I can choose a diet specifically designed for my problem area.
False. It is impossible to lose fat from one part of the body and nowhere else. You lay down your fat cells at three stages of your life (*see* page 48). Whether or not you fill them up depends on what you eat and if you exercise or not. This you can change, but *no* diet can only empty fat from certain cells and not others – it's a physiological impossibility. You will lose fat from where you store it. So if you store fat on your stomach and you diet, that is where you will lose it from.

If I don't eat all day and just have one meal in the evening I will lose weight.
False. In order to keep the metabolic rate elevated, we need to eat regular meals three times a day or more, depending on the amount we eat in one meal. By only eating once in 24 hours, your body is having to conserve fuel for long periods of time. To lose weight, however, you want to get rid of extra fuel quickly. The evening is the worst time to eat your largest meal, as your body slows right down. It is much better to

eat your main meal in the middle of the day, as this is the time when the metabolism is higher because you are moving about. There is also another potential problem with only eating one meal per day: you are far more likely to eat more in one go than you would normally do if you were having three meals per day. The bottom line is that if you eat more calories than you burn, you will store those extra calories as fat. Many people who eat one meal per day tend to pick and snack throughout the day on chocolate bars and biscuits, as they are under the illusion that they are not eating much. All of these habits are more likely to increase your total calorific intake throughout the day one way or another, which means more fat.

Diet pills are a safe and effective way to lose weight.
False. There are so many pills available without a prescription that it's hard to believe that, at the time of printing, there are no enforceable legal requirements these companies have to adhere to. As long as they say 'as part of a calorie controlled diet' and don't promise to do the job all by themselves, almost anything can be sold over the counter. Many of these drugs act on the central nervous system, and have potentially harmful and unpleasant side effects. A friend of mine was placed on a 'metabolism booster' drug, which gave her hallucinations, violent head-aches and insomnia. After a week on the drugs she

looked and felt awful and was unable to continue taking them. For those who do persevere, however, these drugs can be addictive. Appetite suppressants – or any other drugs associated with weight loss – should only be taken by clinically obese patients, when prescribed by their doctor. Even in these circumstances, however, it is still a very controversial area, with a lot of researchers saying that they shouldn't be used at all. There is a difference between foods that are advertised as helping you lose weight as part of a calorie-controlled diet, such as many diet drinks (remember, water will help you lose weight as part of a calorie-controlled diet!), and slimming products, such as those that promise to reduce your appetite.

If I just eat high-protein foods and limit my carbohydrate intake I will lose weight.

False. High-protein diets are, unfortunately, very popular at the moment. As you have learnt from the nutrition section, however, we actually need less protein than any other nutrient. Not only do we not need excess protein, if we take in higher amounts than necessary over a long period of time, we can damage our digestive process. The protein we eat is broken down in the stomach by acids, while all other foods pass through the stomach relatively unchanged and are broken down in the intestines. Eating more protein means we produce more acid, and if the delicate balance between acid and alkaline in the body is disrupted, it can cause digestive disorders. Excess protein, like any other food eaten in excess, is also converted into fat and stored by the body.

I can get rid of excess fat by rubbing in cellulite creams.
False. This is one of the biggest myths of all – where is the fat supposed to go? I don't see it oozing out of the pores and running down legs! No, it stays exactly where it is. Of course any kind of massage is good for the circulation, but your fat cells will only release fat into the blood stream to be burnt as fuel if the body needs it. The only way you can achieve this with a massage cream is if you jump up and down at the same time and continue to rub for 20 minutes or more, so that you stimulate your aerobic energy system into burning fat. A very expensive work-out!

JUST WHAT ARE WE MADE OF?

We are all different. Each individual has a slightly different body composition, which can be divided into three elements: bone, muscle and fat. We often use the term 'Lean Body Mass' (LBM), which means the combined weight of the bones and the muscles added together. The remaining percentage would therefore be classified as fat.

One of the most common reasons people give me

for being overweight is 'I have heavy bones.' Unfortunately for them, they have been misled. Bones are actually incredibly light – as strong as cast iron, but as light as pinewood. It is the fat and the muscle attached to the skeleton that determines our weight, not the size of our bones.

SO WHO'S 'OVERWEIGHT'?

'Overweight' doesn't necessarily mean 'over fat'; they are two completely separate things. Muscle tissue (which makes up most of our LBM) is an active tissue which burns calories in order to stay healthy. Even when at rest, muscles are still burning calories. Fat, on the other hand, does not need any calories; it just sits in its storage sites, stockpiling and doing nothing. Muscles are very heavy, much heavier than fat. This means that we can carry more weight in muscle and not be 'fat', even though the scales tell us we are heavier.

Imagine someone with a similar build to Arnold Schwarzenegger. A very large percentage of his body is muscle, and he carries very little, if any, excess fat. If he used a traditional height/weight chart, however, it would probably tell him that he was overweight. This is because such charts do not account for the fact that muscle is heavier than fat. Therefore, although according to the chart he may be overweight, he certainly isn't over fat.

Similarly, I have a very good friend, Carol, who is a fitness teacher. She is six feet two inches tall and weighs almost thirteen stone. This may sound a lot, but because her body has a large percentage of muscle and a relatively low percentage of fat, she is not over fat. So again, although a height/weight chart may tell her she is overweight, she looks fantastic and turns heads wherever she goes.

As you can see from these examples, the scales do not always tell the whole story. What we need to look at is the body composition, not just the total weight.

EXERCISE IS EVERYTHING

If you don't exercise, your body composition will alter over the years, even if you don't change your eating habits at all. As I've already said, muscle is an active tissue which is designed to be used – to support the skeleton and to enable us to move. All the time we are using our muscles we maintain the same LBM. If we stop using them, however, or use them less, they will literally start to waste away. The individual muscle fibres become smaller and so require less fuel to function. This means, quite simply, that we then need to eat less.

Compare this to the engine in a car. Imagine a large estate car with a very powerful engine. This engine would need a lot of fuel. You may get as little as 20 miles per gallon from this engine, so the tank needs to be very large. Let's say this car's petrol tank holds 12 gallons. Now imagine a small hatchback with a much smaller, less powerful engine. This engine requires less petrol and you may get as much as 40 miles to the gallon out of the car. As a result, there's no need to put in as much petrol and the tank doesn't need to be as big. It may hold a maximum of 8 gallons, so if you tried to put in 12 it would overflow.

Now let's compare this to our muscles. Muscles that are constantly being used require lots of energy, i.e. food, for which they have large storage tanks within the muscle itself. These tanks are constantly being emptied and refilled. On the other hand, muscles that are not constantly used become smaller. They literally shrink and their storage tanks shrink accordingly. So what happens if we try to put in the same amount of fuel as we would in our large muscles? It overflows. The body has a very effective way of mopping up this overflow – it takes the left-over fuel and stores it as fat.

Take a 21-year-old, for example, with a total body weight of 120lb/54kg:

Age	Total Weight	Fat Weight	LBM	% Fat
20	120lb/54kg	26lb/12kg	94lb/43kg	22%

The amount of muscle (i.e. LBM) will determine how much food the body needs in order to function efficiently. If we lose muscle through lack of exercise, therefore, we should reduce the amount of food we eat accordingly. If we don't, as we get older, we will be eating more than our body requires and creating a surplus. This surplus will be stored as fat.

Now let's look at the same woman – who has not exercised – 15 years later, to see what's happened to her body composition:

Age	Total Weight	Fat Weight	LBM	% Fat
35	125lb/57kg	38lb/17kg	87lb/39kg	30%

Her total weight has increased by only 5lb/2kg. Over a 15-year period, most people would be quite happy with a weight increase of this amount. But take a look at her body composition. Because she hasn't exercised, she has *lost* a total of 7lb/3kg of muscle tissue. As muscle requires on average 40 calories per lb/0.4kg per day, she should have reduced her total food intake by 280 calories (i.e. 7 x 40). Since she has continued to eat the same amount as she did when she had 94lb/43kg of muscle, she has overfilled the storage tanks of her muscles and the excess has been stored as fat. This has increased her fat percentage by eight per cent, which would have a dramatic effect on her appearance (it would probably result in an increase of two dress sizes).

PUTTING THE FAT AWAY

Fat is essential. We all need a certain amount of fat in order to protect our organs, and it also forms a vital part of many hormones, our brain and many other cells. We all have essential fat. There is, however, a marked difference between the way in which men and women store their fat.

Women were originally 'designed' to be able to reproduce, and so Mother Nature gave us extra storage sites for fat – on the breasts, hips and thighs – to be readily available to supply all the nutrients required to nourish a growing baby when required. Unfortunately, Mother Nature was rather indiscriminate when dishing out these supplies, and didn't account for the fact that not all women choose to have children, nor for the fact that after we've had our family, we don't need these extra stores any more. Many women struggle for years to get rid of a 'bulge' that is, in fact, specifically designed to be there. They just don't understand why they can't get rid of it. The truth is, we can reduce these 'bulges' quite drastically, but if that's where our fat cells are laid down, we can never eliminate them completely.

What you eat and whether or not you exercise are

not the only factors that determine how you look; genetics also plays a key role. It is generally accepted that we lay down or fill our fat cells at three stages in our life. The first stage is in the womb, and obviously we have no control over that! This is dependent on the genetic make-up we have been given by our parents. The second stage is during the first 12 months of life. Again, this is outside our individual control and dependent on what we are fed. The third and final stage, however, takes place during the 'growth spurt' years, usually our early teens. This we do have more control over – but how many of us really thought that far ahead when we were spending our dinner money on a bag of chips and a can of coke? (Recent research has also shown that obese patients can stimulate the fat cells to multiply further.)

So, while many of us reach adulthood unhappy about the way we look, we think we can change a pattern that has taken years to develop in just a few weeks or months. No, changing body composition permanently takes time, dedication and acceptance of what you are realistically able to achieve.

If, during all three stages, we have laid down more fat cells than are necessary (remember some fat is essential), it doesn't mean that they have to be filled with fat. Think of your fat cells as tiny sacks which take up almost no room at all when they are empty, but lots of room when they are full. If you look at your mother and see that she stores most of her fat on her thighs, then the chances are that you will too. However, you don't have to store as much. That will depend on what you eat and how much you exercise. Genetics will determine where your fat cells are laid down – but *you* determine what and how much you put in them.

Men, on the other hand, don't need these extra storage sites and are given more muscle instead. On average, men store ten per cent less fat than women. It doesn't seem fair does it! Well, it's not all bad news for women. In fact, men are the ones who get the worst deal when it comes to the really important issue of health. Women store more fat on their thighs and less around the abdominal cavity, which is where men tend to store most of their fat. Because this area is much closer to the heart and other vital organs, fatty deposits are more likely to interfere with circulation. This could explain the increased rate of heart attacks in men up to the age of 50, as compared to the statistics in women of the same age. Studies have shown that if men have a waist measurement larger than their hip measurement, their risk of heart disease is increased.

After menopause, however, women's fat deposition sites change, as there is no longer a need for the extra storage on the thighs. Women then begin to store it around the abdominal area, the same as men. (Think about how often you see old ladies with quite skinny legs and a really rounded tummy.) Along with this change comes the increased risk of heart disease, which is much more common in post menopausal women. We also produce less oestrogen – which has a protective effect prior to menopause – so women become as 'at risk' as men.

There have been many theories as to why women have evolved in the way they have, including the 'Stone Age Theory'. The body has an essential need for fuel which comes from the foods we eat – it's common sense. In this day and age, most of us are fortunate enough to live in an environment where the food supply is never in question. We always know that at the end of the day food is available. If we take a look back at how we evolved, however, we see that it wasn't always quite so simple.

Imagine a typical Stone-Age couple, let's call them Mr and Mrs Flintstone. Mr Flintstone didn't go off to the office every morning with his packed lunch, leaving Mrs Flintstone at home to look after the baby and do the baking. He went off, club in hand, to catch and kill supper. Unfortunately for him, however, he wasn't always successful. Some days he may have come home with food and other days with nothing. Mr Flintstone was always the first in line in the food queue; after all, if he wasn't fed, he wouldn't have the energy to go out and catch the next day's supper. Children probably came next in line, with good old mum bringing up the rear and getting whatever was left over. So life went on, with dad using up his fuel chasing around after the next meal, the children using up their fuel in order to grow and develop, but there being often very little left by the time the food finally got around to mum.

As a result, mum became very efficient at storing extra fuel, just in case she had to go without for a while, or in case she became pregnant, so that she would have some fuel in order to nourish a growing baby. It was nature's way of ensuring the continuation of the species! Unfortunately for us, however, nature hasn't realized that some of us have a well-established food supply, and therefore don't need these extra deposits.

Of course this is only one of several theories, but if you are serious about wanting to change your body shape, you must first look around you at your family and your own history of diet and activity levels. Using this information you can then set yourself a *realistic* goal (*see* Chapter 3). The most important benefits you will achieve from this book – if you follow the recipes and the exercises – are the benefits to your *health*. You will have more energy, you will be stronger, your circulation will improve (which may improve your skin and your hair), and you will be able to really live life to the full, and probably live longer. You *will* also lose fat and this will change how you look – but that is an added bonus. *Think Health First.*

Chapter 3

Mind over Matter

The Psychology of Dieting

WHY DO WE DIET?

Most people diet because they want to change the way they look. For whatever reason, we have expectations that our lives would change if we could only lose weight.

Before you begin this programme, I recommend that you sit down quietly and ask yourself exactly what you want to achieve by losing weight. Prioritize your reasons. After all, you may find it very difficult to make some of the long-term changes which are going to be necessary to lose body fat. If you *are* going to make changes, you need a reason for doing so – a specific reason.

THE 'FAT TO FLAT' PLAN

I would encourage you to keep a small book, or a few pages in your diary, devoted to this plan. This will be *your* plan. In it you will individualize all the information I have given you, which will enable you to implement that information in order to achieve your goal.

BEFORE YOU START

You need to start your plan by listing all the things that are important in order for you to achieve your goal, such as shopping, cooking and exercise. You can start to evaluate in your mind things that are *important*. For example, making time to go shopping is *important*; it reduces the risk of being hungry without any food in the house, which could then lead to a fish and chips supper! Exercise is *important*; it helps to burn calories, not just while you are working out, but for the rest of the day. Having an ice cream, however, is definitely *not* important to the success of your diet!

Now try to identify short-term and long-term goals. For example, if you are saving for a new car, the long-term goal is a car. That's all right, but it's a very vague goal, you need to be more specific. Imagine your *favourite* car, one that you could re-alistically afford if you saved, perhaps a blue 1.4 Ford

Escort estate or a green Jaguar. Each time you are tempted to spend money, on a new outfit or a night out, for example, you have to ask yourself what you want more – the outfit/meal or the car. Of course it is possible to have the occasional night out and still get the car; it will just take you a little longer.

The first and most important step towards setting your goal is to be realistic. You have to be able to *achieve* whatever goals you set yourself, not just with regard to weight loss, but with any aspect of your life that you want to change. We are all under intense media pressure to conform to certain images. Every time we open a magazine or a newspaper it seems we are faced with numerous images of 'The Body Beautiful'. But how realistic is that image? It certainly isn't the 'norm', it actually represents the minority.

Think for a moment of all of the people you see regularly, at home or at work. Try to estimate how many people you are thinking of. Now think how many of them have what you would classify as a 'perfect body'. Is it the majority or the minority? Of those with supposedly 'perfect bodies', how many have achieved them by careful eating and regular exercise, and how many were just born lucky?

We all inherit a genetic pattern from our parents. There's nothing we can do about our basic make-up. In fact, approximately 70 per cent of our body composition is pre-determined. That leaves us 30 per cent that we can manipulate, which *can* make a significant difference. As individuals, however, we also have limitations which we must accept.

Unfortunately, this is not recognized by the media. In virtually every aspect of life we are constantly being reminded that 'thin is in'. How would Marilyn Monroe have coped if she was an actress today? I suspect she would have succumbed to the pressures and enlisted the help of a personal trainer and a chef! In adolescent girls particularly, the dissatisfaction with weight is so common that it has become the norm. Many young girls think of their bodies as ugly and despicable and constantly try to hide them, fearing others will view them with hostility and contempt if they are less than perfect. It makes no difference whether they are talented or intelligent – weight is their only concern. They feel that they will be judged by their size alone.

Self acceptance is crucial – we are who we are. Before you start this programme, sit down and write a list of things you like about yourself that have nothing to do with your body image. If you find this difficult, get a close friend to do it for you. Add this to your plan and keep it in a safe place. This will be *very* important for you during times of stress.

Next, write a list of things which you *think* will change in your life when you achieve your target weight loss. Are these things realistic? Do you think

people will like you more? Perhaps you think someone tall, dark and handsome will fall in love with you
and carry you off into the sunset, or that you will get
instant promotion at work. You need to be realistic
and acknowledge that such things are very unlikely
to happen simply because you look more beautiful.

If wonderful things do start to happen to you once
you've lost weight, it's far more likely to be because
of changes in your personality, such as increased
confidence and self-respect. You are more likely to
take greater care of your appearance when you have
a figure which you are happy with. Your attitude to
various issues will change. You may find that you
become a more positive person. Real friendship, however, will not change with the scales; it doesn't go up
as your weight goes down.

Are you *really* ready to undertake this programme? How serious are you about losing weight?
When setting your goals, you must take into account
your current situation. If you are currently in a stress-
ful situation – like moving house, changing jobs or
having problems with relationships – this is probably
not the best time for you to try to lose weight. You are
less likely to succeed, and that in itself may lead to
feelings of depression and frustration.

Overweight people are often described as 'jolly',
but also as frequently suffering from feelings of
inferiority and a deep need to be loved. Whilst this is

true of some overweight people, it is also true of others who have absolutely no need or desire to lose weight. It has been said that obesity (being 30 per cent or more above the maximum desirable weight for each individual) is a way of handling a poor relationship with oneself. This view has now changed, and poor relationships are more often contributed to by the prejudice and discrimination often shown to individuals who are overweight, and *not* the condition itself.

SETTING YOUR GOALS

What is a goal? It is an ultimate aim, a reason for trying. The first thing you need to do is to set yourself a goal for today. Write it down *now*. If it's not written down it's not a goal – it's a dream. Next set yourself a goal for one week (you don't have to start on a Monday, any day will do!) Set additional goals for one month, three months, six months and twelve months. Keep this list of goals somewhere safe, as part of your plan. As you achieve each one, cross it off.

The scales are not the only measure of progress. Go to your local surgery and get the nurse to check your blood pressure and your pulse rate before you start this programme. These are important indicators of fitness, even though they are non-visible. After three months, go back and have them done again, and keep a record of your achievements in your plan. Go back again after six months and one year, to see if you are maintaining your initial improvements. Write these dates in your diary now, as you see the dates creeping up you'll be encouraged to keep up the good work. We all want to do well when we are having a test done, especially if it's going to measure our progress.

I recently went to a talk on motivation which was truly inspirational. The speaker, Mikki Williams, gave each one of us in the room a rubber band to wear around our wrist, just like the ones you get at swimming pools with a locker number on. This band was to represent our goal for the week. When we achieved our goal, we were to take the band off. The results were surprisingly successful. Speaking to others who wore the band, I found that most people did actually keep it on until they achieved their goal, as it served as a reminder that they had a specific objective for that week. Nothing had changed, their *ability* to achieve their goal certainly hadn't changed, but their *desire* to take off the band did inspire them to accomplish their goal.

You could do the same thing. All you need is a thick elastic band. Tell yourself that the band is the reason you are eating less and exercising more. Don't take it off until you have achieved your daily goal each day for one week. Alternatively, how often do you say, 'I don't have time to exercise.' Try putting the band on and not removing it until you have exercised in some form or another at least twice that week. At the start of the following week put it on and do the same thing again. You can use the band as often as you need to. Some people might need to wear it regularly, others may find it useful to wear for a week occasionally, particularly if they think they are going to be in a difficult situation. You may, for example, have several social functions to attend, and the thought of all those profiteroles is just too much to bear, even before you've left home! Make a deal with yourself: 'While I wear this band, not one profiterole will pass my lips.' It will give you a reason for not having one, *try it*, it's surprisingly successful – it really does work.

Having established your goal of wanting to change your body composition and lose fat, there are several factors you should consider before you set a 'target weight'. First of all, what is the lightest weight you have ever maintained for 12 months? Secondly, are you prepared to make the changes necessary in order to lose the weight? You should take into account your current situation. If you are suffering from stress at home or at work, your chances of achieving success may be lessened, and you should take this into account. Be realistic about the changes you can make; they won't happen overnight, and there are several stages in actually changing behaviour patterns.

CHANGE YOUR BEHAVIOUR FOR GOOD

The first stage in changing behaviour patterns is to contemplate change, but you will have already done that if you have bought this book. The next is to prepare, and that is what you are doing now as you read this. You are now acquiring knowledge which – if properly applied – will help you to achieve your goal, knowledge such as what type of exercise you should do and what foods you should eat. Then there is the third stage – action. This involves implementing the changes to your lifestyle, starting to exercise regularly and cooking with less fat, for example. Lastly, there is maintenance. Perhaps surprisingly, this can often be the hardest stage. There are, however, several methods you can use to help you maintain your goal which we will look at.

This strategic plan, from contemplation to maintenance, can be used in almost any situation – it reminds me of when I need to sort out my wardrobe! I spend a few weeks (sometimes months!) thinking what a mess the cupboard is every time I go to get anything out. I promise myself that I *will* tidy it up. Then I try to plan a time when I will be able to do it, such as a quiet day or evening when the family are not around to interrupt me. When this time arrives I take action! Everything comes out. I fill a bag for the next jumble sale, organize what's left and put it away. Full of resolve I determine not to let it get in such a mess again, but maintaining my new method of 'trousers on the left, skirts on the right' soon gets forgotten as the weeks and months go by. It may seem like a strange analogy, but the principles are the same. Deciding to lose weight and to exercise is the easy part! Actually doing it and maintaining it is the hardest.

One of the reasons for this difficulty is that we have to eat. It's not like giving up alcohol – you can't completely abstain from food because if you did you'd die! If you don't eat enough you will be depriving your body of essential nutrients, which it needs in order to be able to function properly. It is very important to accept that we need sufficient nutrients in order for our bodies to function – and that means food.

When you need to lose weight, it is likely you are going to have to give up certain foods which you like. You may find this quite difficult initially, until you experiment and replace them with lower fat alternatives. But you can't just completely give up eating. This means that you have to learn to cope with the situations and foods which, in the past, have caused you to become overweight. But at least these changes have come from your own decision. Imagine, for example, diabetic patients who are suddenly told that they will have to make drastic alterations to their diet. It is much harder for them because that is *enforced* change, whereas at least you have made a conscious decision that you *want* to change. Nevertheless, you will have to cope with various problems in order to achieve and maintain a loss in weight.

You need to develop an overall plan which will enable you to succeed. Then examine how much time and effort is going to be involved in implementing your plan and how it is going to affect other people around you. How much time and effort is it going to take? Will it impede on other important areas of your life, such as family or work commitments? What will the emotional cost be? Is it going to affect your self-esteem? All these questions need to be addressed before you start.

KEEPING SCORE AND STAYING ON TRACK

You will also need to constantly re-evaluate your plan and to adapt it where necessary, depending on how successful you are at achieving your goals. Think of it like a cash-flow forecast for your business, which examines the outgoings and the incomings, to tell you whether or not the accounts will balance at the end of the day. If there is more going out than coming in, you know you need to make changes and alterations to certain elements of the plan, to cut back on certain things in order to meet the repayments. In the same way, if you are not losing weight you will also need to cut back on certain things, such as food, and to increase others, such as exercise. In this way the plan should be constantly adapted to suit you, and those around you. If it's not tailored to meet your individual needs, you are unlikely to stick to it.

If you are not reaching your targets despite eating the right foods (and not eating the wrong ones!) and exercising regularly, you may need to re-evaluate your original expectations. Every individual is different; I cannot give you a target that everyone will be able to reach. What I *can* give you are realistic guidelines. These are that you should be able to lose between ½–2lb/0.2–1kg of body fat per week, *if* you follow the menus and exercise programmes. If you lose more than 2lb/1kg per week it won't all be fat, most of the excess will be fluid. That's because the carbohydrate we eat helps us to store water, so if we cut down on the amount of carbohydrate we eat, we are naturally going to lose some fluid. Once this new level has been established, the rate of loss will probably slow down to within the levels I have stated. You should take this information into account when evaluating your achievements on the scales.

YOU'RE NOT ALONE

When designing your plan it is also important to ask the people around you for support. Consider how your actions are going to affect them. Perhaps someone else in the family will have to prepare the evening meal occasionally, to give you time to attend an exercise class or to exercise at home. If you set the guidelines before you start, there needn't be any unpleasant surprises for anyone.

Equally as important is to establish that your plan doesn't mean that everyone will be on hunger rations for the next few months! The changes you make when cooking don't have to affect the rest of the family. You will be able to eat many of the same foods as before, even though some will need to be prepared differently. It is, however, possible for the whole family to be put on a low-fat highly nutritious diet and not even know it (*see* page 27). *Remember, a diet doesn't necessarily have to mean 'losing weight', a healthy diet can mean just eating more healthily.*

WHEN TEMPTATION STRIKES

Within your plan you should also have strategies
for coping with temptation or relapses. It is asking
a lot to expect yourself to be able to suddenly give
up chocolate, cheese, ice cream, or whatever your
favourite high-fat foods are. Write down your
favourite high-fat foods. Then write down exactly
what it is you like about them. At first you'll probably
say everything! But you need to analyse your feelings
and be specific. Is it the colour, the texture, the taste,
the feeling you get when you're eating it, or the feeling you get when you've finished it? Then write
down what you are usually doing when you eat these
foods. This may vary from time to time, but you may
be surprised to see a pattern forming.

Now ask yourself exactly what it is you are
getting from these foods. Are you eating to satisfy
feelings of hunger (in which case you've just been
making wrong choices), or is it to relieve boredom,
such as while watching television, or do you comfort
eat to relieve tension? Late night snacks can become
a habit, so rather than trying to stop having one
altogether (which will leave you feeling deprived),
try having a healthier option instead. Prepare some
nibbles *before* you feel peckish. Vegetables with a
yogurt-based dip, for example, can be a very tasty
low-fat alternative to crisps and peanuts. I often

make a large bowl of fresh fruit salad and dip into it whenever I am hungry. One of my favourite evening snacks is a bowl of cornflakes mixed with fresh fruit salad and semi-skimmed milk. Cereal can also be a low-calorie, low-fat snack for any time of the day. Of course, if you are trying to lose weight, it is better not to have a late night snack at all but, if you must have something, choose carefully.

'I only wanted one, but once I'd opened the packet I had to finish it; I couldn't help myself, I lost control.' How familiar does this sound? What is this word 'control', that we all seem to lack from time to time? The dictionary defines it as: 'power to direct or determine'. We *do* ultimately have the control, or power, to determine whether or not we will have one biscuit, or the packet. Imagine your favourite high-fat food, perhaps a piece of chocolate cake. Picture yourself sitting in front of the cake, with a strong desire to eat it. If I told you that it was made with salt instead of flour, and that even one bite would make you violently sick, would you still want to eat it? Probably not! But if you had *really* lost control, you would *have* to eat it, no matter what. The fact is, we don't lose control at all, we just choose not to exercise our control at a particular moment.

Visualizing yourself *not* eating foods which you will have to give up, or at least cut down on, can be a very good way of preparing yourself for facing unavoidable difficult situations – such as social gatherings, where you know tempting foods will be available. Visualize your host offering you a tempting selection of cheese and you saying 'No thank you.' Ponder this image several times, varying the situation and the food. It may sound a little strange, but positive imagery is very powerful. Think of world-class runners waiting for the start of the race ahead. Are they standing around chatting? Certainly not, they are busy concentrating, imagining running as fast as possible and breaking the tape, imagining and positively visualizing success. You, too, can imagine *your* success, it will help you to believe you *can* do it.

Handling High-Risk Situations

For real long-term success, you need to be able to identify 'high-risk' situations – some predictable and some not – which will undoubtedly come along. You will have two choices, each leading to a very different outcome, both in the short term and the long term:

A. High-Risk Situation
↓
No 'coping' skills
↓
Initial lapse in eating pattern
↓
Decreased confidence
↓
Loss of 'control'

In this example, you don't have the skills to avoid the foods you know you should not be eating. You will, as I have mentioned, undoubtedly come across a wide range of circumstances where you are tempted to deviate from your plan. If you do not know how to handle high-risk situations, you are likely to experience a short-term lapse, which may snowball into completely abandoning your plan altogether. This inevitably leads to decreased confidence, and to eating more than you did before you went on the 'diet' in order to 'cheer yourself up', thereby making the problem worse than it was in the first place

So what is *coping?* Coping is being able to identify high-risk situations, and to develop ways of dealing with those risks. First, and most importantly, you have to recognize what is 'high risk' for you – this will vary according to your likes and dislikes. If possible, avoid the situation altogether, in order to prevent the problem occurring. This doesn't necessarily mean never going out; it just means pre-planning. For example, if you have been invited to a friend's house for a meal, you *must* tell your host that you are avoiding high-fat foods. You don't even have to use the word 'diet'. After all, if you are a vegetarian or allergic to a certain food, I'm sure you don't hesitate to mention this, knowing that your host *won't* mind, as his/her aim is to prepare a meal that you are going to enjoy – not one that makes you feel guilty and depressed after you've eaten it.

If you're eating out at a restaurant, you need to be aware of the kind of food the restaurant serves *before* you go. If they only offer foods in rich, creamy (fatty) sauces, then try phoning before you go to ask if they would prepare you something that is not on the menu. Most places will be happy to do this – if not, choose another restaurant (*see* page 33 for advice on eating out).

Alternatively, you may be tempted to go out for the meal and not say anything, to just have a 'night off'. This means giving yourself permission to eat all the foods you have been trying so hard to avoid. If you do this once, you will find yourself doing it again and again, and your resolve and determination will decrease rapidly. Do you want to lose willpower or weight?

With a little bit of pre-planning, you should be able to enjoy the same social patterns as you did before you started your weight-loss plan. If you start to decline invitations, you are depriving yourself of something that you previously enjoyed, and this can lead to feelings of resentment – not just for you, but for partners and friends as well. In order to succeed on this plan you must try and make the minimum number of changes to your normal social activities, otherwise you are unlikely to stick to it.

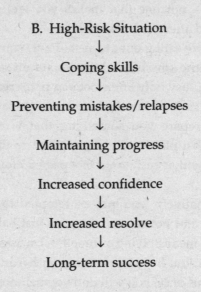

B. High-Risk Situation
↓
Coping skills
↓
Preventing mistakes/relapses
↓
Maintaining progress
↓
Increased confidence
↓
Increased resolve
↓
Long-term success

In this second example, you have developed the skills and tactics to enable you to handle the high-risk situations. As you can see, the end result is very different from the first example. The situation was exactly the same, you just handled it differently at a very early stage. It may take you some time to develop the skills we have talked about in this section, but they are *crucial* to long-term success.

It is also important to recognize that if you do lapse, it doesn't mean you have 'failed'. If you lose one battle, you won't necessarily lose the war! However, it *will* weaken your defences, so get straight back on the plan and determine not to do it again.

Exercise also plays a vital role in helping you to stick to the plan. Many studies have shown that people who exercise have higher self-esteem and are less likely to suffer from stress. Because exercise is a positive habit (something that you *do*), it makes you feel better. Dieting, on the other hand, is associated with negative feelings and things that you *can't do* – 'I can't eat cheese', 'I can't eat chocolate', for example. The good news is the more you exercise, the less you focus on the negative aspects. The longer you stick to the plan, the more your physical image will change and your confidence increase. And as low-fat, controlled eating and regular exercise become part of your life, so will your improved shape and health become part of your life, too. That has to be worth working for!

I hope this has given you some valuable information that you will use to develop your own coping skills. Whenever you are faced with a difficult situation and are able to control it, write it down in your diary or in your plan in big bold letters – as a reminder that you *can* do it. On the other hand, if you have tried something that hasn't worked, make a mental note of it, and next time you are faced with a similar situation try a different tactic. You will soon develop your own ways and means. Remember, it is impossible to lose control, you just choose not to exercise control in certain situations – it's up to you.

Chapter 4

Fat – The Vital Statistics

Everything You Need to Know about Fat

How much do you know about fat? Most people think of fat as the excess we store on our body, but there is much more to it than that. The fat we store on our body isn't the same as the fat we eat, although some people think that if they eat a cream cake it will go straight to their thighs! Well, it is true that it sometimes ends up there, but it is not a direct route.

THE FAT WE EAT

The fat we eat is made up of fatty acids which are bonded together to form long chains. Once these chains have been broken, the fatty acids can be digested. The difference between saturated and unsaturated fats is the way in which the fatty acids are held together in their chains. Saturated fats are held together by single bonds. They are usually of animal origin and are *solid* at room temperature. These are the fats which we should avoid, as they are associated with an increased risk of heart disease and possibly cancer. Unsaturated fats are usually of vegetable origin and are held together by double bonds. They are *liquid* at room temperature and include both polyunsaturated and monounsaturated fats.

Unsaturated fats often turn rancid when oxygen breaks down the bonds, causing a harmful chain reaction which releases free radicals. Preservatives – in the form of antioxidants – are added to prevent this from occurring. Antioxidants attach themselves to the free radicals so that they become disabled and cannot cause any damage. Some vitamins, zinc and selenium are antioxidants. Many natural antioxidants can be found in green, leafy vegetables, which should therefore be eaten regularly.

Scientists and chemists are able to change the structure of fat. Many of the spreads we buy contain hydrogenated fat – unsaturated fat that has been treated to make it become solid at room temperature, thereby enabling us to use it as a spread. This was supposed to have the health benefits of unsaturated fat with the spreading ability of saturated fat. Unfortunately, however, research is now showing that serious health hazards can occur as a result of this process and that hydrogenated fats should be avoided. Many processed foods, including crisps, also contain hydrogenated fats – another good reason for not eating them!

PUTTING FAT TO WORK FOR ENERGY

Fat is a great energy provider: per gram, it gives us far more energy than carbohydrate. Our bodies are designed to make optimum use of this 'wonderfuel'. A typical male can store about 150k in carbohydrate and a typical female 164k, which is enough to last approximately two days – but we have the ability to store *billions* of calories of potential energy in the form of fat. We also have a specialized system which enables us to store fat within the fat cells. If we had to store carbohydrate in the same way, we would all be huge, as every gram of carbohydrate also stores four grams of water. Our ability to move around would be severely limited and we'd probably take up a room each! Thankfully, nature has given us a far more practical solution – so the next time you're thinking how large your thighs look because they store fat, just consider how much larger they'd be if you had to store carbohydrate!

Unfortunately, we cannot burn all this potential fat as energy without carbohydrate. Think, for example, of a marathon runner at the end of a race, totally exhausted because he has used up all his carbohydrate stores. Although he has billions of calories of fat energy left, he can't get to them – how frustrating! This means that you'll be disappointed if you go onto a very low-calorie diet in the belief that you will be burning lots of fat from your reserve supplies. If you are not taking in regular supplies of carbohydrate, your body is unable to burn the fat, no matter how much or how little you have. Carbohydrate is like the key that unlocks the door to the fat cell. You must eat properly if you want to lose fat. Very low-calorie diets will not be providing the amount of carbohydrate you need. They will also dramatically reduce the amount of water you store (1 gram of carbohydrate stores 4 grams of water), which means that your total body weight will drop drastically, even though you have lost little or no fat (*see* pages 44–7).

FROM YOUR FOOD TO YOUR FIGURE

So how does the fat we eat become fat we store? The body is full of enzymes which help us to break down our food. The enzyme responsible for breaking down fat and transporting it to the blood is called lipase. Lipoprotein lipase is a long chemical arm that sits in the blood vessel and latches onto passing fat. It opens the door to the fat cell, throws the fat inside and then shuts the door. This enzyme can work very quickly or very slowly, according to how much practice it gets. Like all the body's systems, it can be trained to be more effective. If it is constantly bombarded with high levels of fat in the blood, it will work much harder and faster to take it out of the blood and put it into the fat cells, filling them up and making us fatter. Fatter people get fatter more easily and more quickly as this system becomes more efficient. The good news is, you *can* do something to change the rate and slow the lipoprotein lipase down, by eating less fat over a long period of time. It is also possible to change taste preferences for fat in just 12 weeks, after which time fatty foods which you previously enjoyed can leave you with a very unpleasant taste in your mouth.

Insulin also stimulates fat storage. Insulin is a hormone secreted by the pancreas which monitors blood sugar levels. If the blood becomes bombarded with very high levels of sugar, insulin is released to escort fat from the blood to the tissues. If you eat foods that are high in sugar *and* high in fat, you are literally training your body to store fat. Ice cream, for example, is just sugar-coated fat. If you eat it – you eventually wear it! If you want to lose body fat, you need to avoid foods that are high in sugar, as well as those that are high in fat.

Fat cells are often called cellulite or adipose tissue. They are *all* fat cells, so don't be tricked by clever marketing. A fat cell is fat by any other name. Fat is constantly being sucked into the fat cells, it is a normal process – everyone is storing fat all the time. We tend to think of fat cells as deposit accounts, where plenty goes in and very little comes out. In fact, our fat cells are constantly sucking in fat and spitting it out; they are active all the time. What determines their size is whether fat is coming in faster than it is going out, or vice versa. Either way, the system can be trained – and changed.

Saturated fats are stored very easily in fat cells. For example, the body finds it easier to store lard as body fat than it does olive oil. So if you eat 1,000 calories of each, although the energy potential is the same (i.e. 1,000 calories), more of the lard is likely to end up in your fat cells than the oil. Overall, fat is more fattening gram per gram than carbohydrate, because the body doesn't have to work very hard to convert it from dietary fat to body fat. Whatever foods you eat, a certain amount of energy provided by that food will be used to break down the food itself. In the case of carbohydrate, approximately 23 per cent of the calories consumed are used up re-packaging it for fat storage. In the case of fat, only 3 per cent of the calories are used to make it suitable for fat storage – so there are more calories left to be stored as fat.

If you eat a high-carbohydrate diet, you are more likely to consume roughly the amount of calories you need. If you eat a high-fat diet, you are almost certainly going to be consuming more calories than you need. It isn't difficult to overeat 800 calories in one meal, if you choose creamy sauces and fatty meats, along with a high-fat dessert. Just think how quickly the calories can add up! On the other hand, it would be very difficult to overeat 800 calories of carrots! The reality is, of course, that so many readily available foods have a very high-fat content. We have to make a conscious effort to read food labels – to see exactly what and how much we are eating – in order to keep our energy requirements roughly equal to our energy intake (what we eat). Many people who think they are eating a healthy diet are actually consuming far more fat than they need.

APPLES AND PEARS

Over recent years there has been a lot of research looking at how and where we store our body fat, particularly at the effects of storing it around the mid-section of the body. Upper-body obesity is far more common in males than females, although it isn't totally sex specific (*see* pages 48–52). The fat cells in the abdominal area have a tendency to spit out their fat when they get too full. The fat then goes into the blood and circulates to the liver. To combat this, more insulin is produced and it becomes a vicious circle. The fat cells which release the second largest amount of fat into the blood are around the buttocks, and the third largest area is around the hips. This would seem to endorse the long-held belief that you lose fat from the top down.

LETTING GO OF FAT

Once the fat has been packaged into the fat cells, it may stay there for some time or be passed out fairly quickly to be used for energy. This will depend on two things; firstly, how much fat you are putting into the cells, and secondly, how much you are taking out to be used for fuel. We have approximately 25–75 billion fat cells, all of which are potentially very active; fat is shuttling in and out all the time.

Fat cells have efficient systems both for storing and releasing fat. If both systems are working at approximately the same rate, you will maintain your current level of body fat. If one system is working faster than the other, you will be either losing or gaining fat. The rate at which fat passes in and out of the cell can vary throughout the day, but overall it will level out at a set rate, according to how you have trained the systems over a long period of time. This is called the 'set point theory'. It means that the fat cells will protect their set rate of taking in and releasing fat – even if you change what you eat or the amount you exercise for a short period of time.

If you have been on a diet in the past and reached a plateau after a few weeks, it may be because your body is trying to protect its set point. However, if you continue to exercise (*see* pages 111-112), you *will* be able to change this set rate and get past the stumbling block in a matter of weeks. So don't lose heart – it's just your body adapting to a new set of circumstances. It is quite natural and very common.

The best way to cope with a plateau is to change something, either what or how much you eat, for example, or to try eating your main meal at lunch time instead of in the evening. It may just mean eating smaller meals more often. We don't have to stick rigidly to the regime of three meals per day. I often go all day 'grazing', particularly in the summer when it's hot. As long as you are aware of the total amount of food you are eating, and don't see it as a licence to eat four or five large meals per day, it may be just what you need to kick-start your body into releasing fat. As every individual is different, you will need to experiment a little, but always allow time for the changes to occur.

Many 'new' dieters experience a rebound effect after about a month, as the body tries to defend its original set point. This is quite normal and should be treated in the same way as a plateau. Exercise also plays a key role. Perhaps you need to change the type of exercise you are doing, or else exercise for longer (*see* page 112 for an exercise plan). Remember, the key to breaking a plateau or a rebound is to introduce *change*.

If your rate of weight loss is very slow, it is likely that the enzyme responsible for releasing fat from the cell is working quite slowly. However, a steady rate of 1lb/0.4kg per week fat loss is considered to be very healthy, and in the long term the weight is more likely to stay off. However slow your progress is, if you are releasing more fat from the cells than you are putting in, you are succeeding in your long-term goal – improving your health and your self-image.

Fat is released from the fat cells using a hormone called Hormone Sensitive Lipase (HSL). This hormone works in the reverse manner to lipoprotein lipase, which puts the fat into the cell. It sits at the edge of the cell and is stimulated by nerves to reach into the cell, scoop out some fat and put it into the blood, where it can be carried off to be burnt as fuel. High insulin levels prevent HSL from functioning efficiently, so eating a high-sugar meal not only enhances your ability to store fat quickly and efficiently, but also 'locks' fat in the cell so that it can't get out. This is a very good reason for not eating ice cream or any other sugar/fat combination. On the other hand, if you want to put fat in your fat cells, it's the best way to do it!

Fat is stored all over the body. We always have fat in the blood readily available for use, and we can also store quite large amounts within the muscles. To improve body composition, however, we need to stimulate the release of fat from the fat cells and into the blood where it can be used up. Exercise is one of the best ways to improve body composition, as the burning of fat takes place in the muscle. In fact, the *only* place where you can burn fat is in the muscle.

By exercising regularly, you can train your body to metabolize more fat more quickly, not just when you are exercising, but *all the time*. It's this process that will really accelerate fat loss. We actually burn relatively little fat whilst we are working out, but because we increase the ratio of lean body tissue to fat mass on the body, we increase the amount of fat and calories we burn every day in just staying alive. If you exercise regularly, you can burn more fat even when you are asleep! That has to be good news. The cruel truth is, if you don't change your habits and you are fat, you will just get fatter. This will have serious implications for your health, as well as affecting how you feel about yourself and the way you look.

It should be noted at this point that you must be careful about restricting a child's intake of fat. This is because fat is vital for providing the sheaths that surround and protect our nerves as we grow and develop. Children up to the age of five should, therefore, have full-cream milk. What you can do, however, is change the quality of the fat they are getting, by restricting saturated fats and encouraging them to eat oily fish and unsaturated fats. Cooking with extra virgin olive oil is much healthier, for example. Rolls with sesame seeds are also an excellent source of natural oils – preferably without a greasy burger in the middle!

Chapter 5

Exercise – Why Bother?

What's in It for You?

Unfortunately, most people don't bother. The Allied Dunbar Survey, conducted in the UK in 1992, showed that although over 80 per cent of people in the UK believe that exercise is good for you, 80 per cent don't exercise. In fact, in the over–55 age group, 50 per cent of women could not stand up from a chair or climb the stairs unaided. These are basic skills necessary to maintain independence. Many studies in the US have shown similar results.

HOW FIT IS FIT?

Some time ago, I toured the country presenting a talk called 'Why Exercise?' to groups consisting mostly of women. I began each talk by discussing the definition of 'fitness' and the different groups came up with their own definitions as to what it actually means. Overall, each group had very similar ideas. These included:

'Being able to get through the day without feeling
shattered.'
'Having enough energy to do the housework *and*
play with the children.'
'Being able to walk to work and use the stairs instead
of the lift.'
'Having enough energy to walk the dog without
getting puffed out.'

All of these are very accurate definitions of fitness
and describe what fitness meant to each individual.
What would your definition of fitness be?

Having discussed the merits of 'being fit', I then
asked the ladies (and some men) to write down the
name of someone they could think of who was fit.
Their suggestions included Linford Christie, Sally
Gunnell, Daley Thompson, Colin Jackson and many
other similar figures. These are all elite athletes,
people who, through very intensive training, have
become the best in the world. I then asked them to
look again at their original definitions of fitness,
and together we went through the list and asked the
questions: 'Were these athletes fit enough to get
through the day without feeling shattered?' 'Could
they walk the dog without getting puffed out?' The
answer to both these questions was clearly 'yes', but,
most importantly, did they actually need to be as
fit as they were in order to do these everyday

things? The answer was, of course, 'no'.

Many people today seem to have the preconceived idea that fitness is something unachievable. When I talk about fitness, I am talking about the following: a body that is healthy enough to be able to withstand disease; a body that can recover quickly from minor illness; a body that allows its owner freedom to complete everyday tasks without the restrictions of breathlessness and discomfort.

The human body is nothing short of a miracle. I have been designing work-outs and studying nutrition for the past 15 years, and yet it *still* astounds me that the body uses so many interrelated and complicated systems in order to function. In addition to this, I have seen people literally change their lives and their health – not to mention their shape – just by training their body and teaching it to improve its efficiency. There is no piece of machinery in the world that has this ability to improve itself by training, but the human body can. The secret is quite simple – to challenge your body to work slightly harder than it does already.

How many of us could recite our 13 times table if asked? I certainly couldn't, because I have only been programmed to recite my tables up to 12. Your body has the same limitations – it will function only according to the demands you place on it and no more. So if you don't exercise regularly and challenge your heart and muscles, they will become smaller and weaker because your body thinks they are not needed. All you need to do to reverse this process is to start to place gentle demands on your body systems. If you do this regularly, the body will get stronger and improve itself to adapt to the new demands. The heart will get stronger and pump more blood, the muscle fibres will get stronger to give you more strength. In fact, muscle fibres can even get longer to allow you more flexibility. It's fantastic!

The good news is that you don't have to work very hard for these miraculous changes to occur. You will, in fact, reap the most benefit in the first few weeks of training. Someone who has never exercised can improve their fitness levels by a staggering 25–35 per cent in the first few weeks. You will start to feel fitter because you will be teaching your body to use more of the oxygen you are breathing in to help provide you with energy.

FINDING YOUR WAY TO EXERCISE

What do you associate the word 'exercise' with? Most people who don't exercise associate it with pain or discomfort. For some, the mere mention of the word sends shivers down their spine, conjuring up visions of cross country-runs and those awful PE knickers that seemed to come up to your chin! Or ankle socks that barely covered your feet and left your legs feeling cold and blue! I can remember several less than pleasant exercise experiences at school: the clunking of hockey sticks that left me with bruises up to my knees; playing wing defence in netball to an attacker who was so much taller than me that she almost trod on me as she went past; spending an hour and a half serving tennis balls into the net, driving my opponent into a rage.

Despite all this, however, I was very fortunate in that even though I hated all the outdoor sports, once I was in the warm and cosy gymnasium – with lovely soft crash mats and lots of ropes and poles to swing around on – I loved it. The result of finding an activity I really enjoyed was that I started to do more of it and, before long, was training regularly and entering competitions. The moral of this story is quite obvious – you have to find some kind of activity that you enjoy or you won't stick to it. You need to choose a form of exercise that you can do without dreading it. If you find something you are good at you will want to do it more – it's human nature. Your motivation will also increase after a month or so, as you start to see and feel the benefits.

You may find that you prefer to exercise with someone else or in a group setting. Have a look in your local paper for details of fitness classes in your area. It doesn't have to be aerobics. There are lots of different types of classes, such as 'Tums and Bums', 'Circuits', or 'Stretch and Tone'. It will not necessarily matter which one you choose – *all* exercise has a very important part to play if you are serious about losing weight.

If you are going to go to an organized class, make sure that the instructor is qualified. In the UK the recognized qualification is RSA Teacher of Exercise to Music (in the US the qualifications are A.F.A.A. or A.C.E.). If the instructor has this, you can be assured that they have undergone at least 80 hours of training, including anatomy, physiology, exercise safety and a written and practical exam. Don't be afraid to ask your instructor about their qualification – if they have one, they will have worked so hard to earn it that they will be only too happy to tell you! Unfortunately, not all teachers who qualify continue to maintain such high standards once they have passed their exam. Do you drive your car in the same way as you did for your driving test? Probably not.

The fitness industry is constantly changing. We are learning more about the body all the time, and as we learn more about how the body adapts to exercise, we are able to design safer training programmes. It is vital, therefore, that instructors keep up-to-date with the latest information. A good instructor will regularly attend seminars and further training courses, to make sure that the information they are giving is correct. Here are a few more guidelines to help you choose a good instructor:

- Did they ask you to complete a health questionnaire before commencing the class?
- Do they regularly check that everyone is all right – no recent injuries or illnesses, for example?
- Does the class always begin with a *gentle* warm-up (you should *never* feel breathless in the warm-up).
- Do they constantly remind you about good technique and posture?
- Do they give good demonstrations of what they want you to do?
- Do they move around to make sure that everyone is doing the exercise correctly, or are they too busy having a work-out themselves?
- Do they help or correct participants who are not in the right position?
- Can you hear the instructions clearly above the music?
- Do they face the class and really look at individuals, as opposed to facing the mirror and watching themselves?
- Do they always offer alternatives for people of varying fitness levels?
- Do you feel that it's the instructor's work-out or your work-out?
- Do they make themselves available for questions

before or after the class, or are they always talking about themselves and what *they* can do?

These are just a few of the qualities to look for when choosing an instructor. Don't be afraid to be choosy; after all, you are literally putting your body in their hands. If you make a bad choice you could end up getting injured.

Of course you don't have to go to an exercise class to have a good work-out. There are lots of other alternatives, and what is on offer in a class may not suit everyone. For example, some people would benefit from activity levels that are non-strenuous or not particularly long in duration. It is certainly not compulsory to experience the 'high' sensation that some people get from exercising to the point of near exhaustion! It's important to remember that *most* people don't actually like the feeling of being hot and sweaty with aching limbs. What they do like, however, is the feeling of satisfaction and wellbeing they experience after they have exercised, a feeling which can last for several hours. You'll find a list of alternatives to classes in the following chapter – choose whatever's right for you.

REAPING THE REWARDS

When I was teaching fitness classes three nights per week, I often used to sit on the sofa half an hour before I was due to leave and wish that I didn't have to go. I used to think 'I can't be bothered.' Does that sound familiar? How many times do *you* make that excuse, or perhaps, 'I'm too tired' or 'I haven't got time'. I am thankful now that I did go, since I have managed to stay healthy and in good shape as a result. You would be amazed at how many people say to me 'You're so lucky to have a figure like that,' when, in fact, luck has little to do with it. It's true that I have never been drastically overweight, but that is because I have always watched what I eat and have exercised regularly. I am as predisposed as most people to gaining weight, particularly as I have grown older (I seemed to age visibly on my 30th birthday!) However, it's not just my figure – my skin and hair really suffer if I eat greasy food and don't work out. I feel grumpy and lethargic and lose the motivation to want to exercise, which, of course, makes the situation worse.

Exercise can help us in so many ways. Weight loss is just one benefit, although it is perhaps the most outwardly visible. There are, however, many psychological benefits including: being better able to cope with stress; being less likely to suffer from depression; being able to recover more quickly from illness – and so the list goes on.

The beauty of exercise is that the benefits are so long lasting. If you work out for an hour in the morning, the benefits you generate will keep on working for hours afterwards. Your metabolic rate will be increased, which means burning more calories – including fat. Your heart and other muscles will be adapting to the new demands and will be making themselves stronger – this also requires more calories. Your circulation and digestive system will also be benefiting, and all this is happening whilst you go about your daily tasks. It reminds me of a recent commercial on television for a mouthwash. In the first shot you see a man getting ready for work, cleaning his teeth and using the mouthwash. A few minutes later, after another advert, up pops the same man supposedly later in the day at work. He smiles and says, 'It's still working.' A few minutes later, after yet another advert, the same man appears in the evening scene with the same comment, 'It's still working.' The benefits are still being achieved hours after the event has taken place – it's exactly the same with exercise.

It's not just the energy cost of the exercise that is important – that is, how many calories you burn up while actually working out – it's how many calories you need to burn just to stay alive. If you are over-weight, there is visible evidence that you are eating more than you need. If you exercise regularly, however, that daily requirement – the number of calories you need to stay alive and healthy – will increase as you replace lost muscle tissue, and you really will burn more calories 24 hours per day, even whilst you sleep! That's one kind of exercise we all have to find time for.

Good health and the prevention of disease are basic human needs. We invest huge sums of money trying to 'buy health', when we actually have most of the answers completely free of charge. With regular exercise you can extend your life span by several years, not to mention drastically improve your quality of life. Think ahead for a moment. If you cannot stand up from a chair unaided, then you cannot get off the toilet unaided. This means that the chances of you living at home and not being institutionalized when you get older are slim, as your muscles and heart will have weakened so much due to inactivity that you will no longer be able to look after yourself. Exercise is not just about losing weight, it is a free prescription for a healthy body.

IT'S NEVER TOO LATE

People often tell me that they are too old to exercise, but that is simply not true. Providing you are in good general health, there is no reason whatsoever why you cannot begin a gentle exercise programme and reap the same benefits as someone younger. There is little or no difference between the improvements gained by elderly people starting exercise programmes and those achieved by people in their 20s.

In a recent study, scientific researchers wanted to test this theory out. They went along to their local residential care centre and asked for some volunteers to start an exercise programme. They were met initially with cries of horror from the staff, but once they'd persuaded them that it was all perfectly safe and that the participants would be very well supervised, they did manage to get a few residents to join in. These residents felt that they had nothing better to do since they were only sitting around waiting to die anyway! The programme began very gently with some mobility work in a chair, and over the course of a few months they progressed to include some strength work, to try to regain some of the muscle tissue lost due to years of inactivity. At the same time, similar exercise programmes were being carried out with college students. The work-outs were adapted to their increased level of fitness and both groups were worked at approximately 80 per cent of their maximum potential.

When the results were compared at the end of the programme, it was noted that the residents had dramatically improved their quality of life. They were more active during the day, they were more likely to play table tennis and go for walks rather than just sit around all day, and their medication requirements had gone down – in some cases, quite drastically. In addition to this, the results of the original test – which was to see whether or not they could gain the same improvements in muscle tissue as the younger students – showed clearly that they had. The replacing of lost muscle tissue was far more significant to the residents than the younger group, because it literally changed their lives. When the researchers completed their study, they were persuaded to stay and design a much larger programme for the other residents, who had seen the changes in those who had taken part and now wanted the same benefits themselves. The oldest resident who took part in the study was apparently in his 90s!

THE RIGHT PROGRAMME FOR YOU

So what is the best form of exercise for you? The answer is very simple – it's the form of exercise which you enjoy doing and which fits in best with your daily routine. If it doesn't fit into your lifestyle without any major changes, you will not stick to it.

In order to work out the best exercise programme for you, you need to decide exactly what you want to achieve by exercising – weight loss, for example. Different types of exercise have different effects on the body, and the exercise programmes in this book have been specifically designed to help you lose weight. I believe you are more likely to stick to the exercise programme if you understand exactly what is going on inside your body whilst you are working out. So let's take a look at the body's energy systems.

It may surprise you to learn that we have several ways of producing the energy required to make our muscles contract, and that not all of them burn fat. The body is able to utilize different foods – such as fat, carbohydrate and protein – in different ways in order to provide us with energy. These foods are the energy nutrients (*see* page 7). Just as we have a choice between which fuels we use in our homes – gas, electricity or both – so the body has two main energy systems to choose from. Which one we use is determined by the following: how many muscles are working; how hard; how fast they are working; and what foods are available to provide the fuel.

THE AEROBIC ENERGY SYSTEM

This is by far the most efficient of the two systems. 'Aerobic' means that the body is using oxygen to help it break down the food molecules which are being used to provide energy. The foods required for this are carbohydrates (which are broken down into glycogen or blood sugar) and fats (which are broken down into fatty acids). Together these go through a series of chemical changes within the muscle, giving it the power to contract.

Unfortunately, we cannot burn fat without glycogen. One of the reasons why so many people fail with low-calorie diets is that they are not eating enough carbohydrate to provide the glycogen necessary to burn fat. They may lose body weight but, as explained in the chapter on body composition (*see* pages 46-7), although they end up weighing less, they have a higher percentage of fat on their body and so look very 'flabby'. As soon as they resume a normal eating pattern, they regain all their lost weight and more.

The aerobic energy system is very similar to gas central heating – it takes a long time to 'get going', but once it does, it is extremely cost effective and the output is very good. It gives us lots of energy for long periods of time, providing we are not working too hard. It is entirely dependent on the efficiency of the cardiovascular system (the heart and circulation) in pumping oxygen around the body and into the cells (inside the working muscles), which break down the fat and glycogen. Examples of the types of activity that use aerobic energy include walking, swimming, jogging and cycling.

Each individual has a different aerobic capability based on the efficiency of their heart and lungs. As soon as the level of the activity becomes too high, the body switches to the anaerobic energy system.

THE ANAEROBIC ENERGY SYSTEM

This second energy system comes into effect when the heart cannot pump oxygen around the body quickly enough. It breaks down glycogen but *not* fat, and it does so without the use of oxygen. We use this system when the need for energy is greater and more immediate. Examples of anaerobic activities include squash, sprinting, high/long jump and other short-term power-based events.

If you came home to a cold house, an electric fan heater would give you more heat more quickly than gas central heating. The anaerobic energy system also gives us more power more quickly. However, the disadvantage is that we cannot keep going at a high level of intensity for very long. The reason for this is that we can only store limited amounts of glucose in the muscle (muscle glycogen), and when this runs out, we have to wait for the liver to process some more and to deliver it to the muscle. On the other hand, with the aerobic energy system the supply of glycogen lasts much longer, because fat is providing most of the fuel and glycogen stores are spared.

HOW HARD SHOULD YOU WORK?

One of the biggest areas of controversy concerns how hard you should work in order to maximize the amount of fat you burn whilst you are working out. The truth is that *whatever* form of exercise you do, you will be helping your body to burn fat, not only whilst you are exercising but all the time. One school of thought is that if you work too hard you *won't* burn fat. This is based on the principle that because it takes a long time for the fat to be taken out of the fat cells, into the blood stream, into the muscle and then finally broken down, you need to exercise for quite a long time in order to stimulate this process. In other words, by the time the fat has been taken to the muscle you will have already finished exercising. There is a lot of scientific evidence to support this and in principle it is true.

To maximize the amount of fat you burn whilst you are working out, you should aim to keep going for longer, to give your fat cells more time to release their fat. You should also remember that if you do this regularly, you will be training your fat cells to release fat into the bloodstream to be used as fuel (*see* pages 84–5). In order to do this, you will need to keep the level of exercise fairly low/moderate – after all, Linford Christie could not run as fast over 1,500 metres as he does over 100 metres. In general terms, you should feel breathless but not exhausted (*see* the activity level scale on pages 113–14).

There are several ways in which you can estimate how hard you are working in order to see whether or not you are burning fat. The first is to take your pulse rate whilst you are at the hardest point of the exercise. The problem with this, however, is that if you are moving about (jogging or swimming, for example) it is almost impossible to take your pulse accurately. You will also need to work out in advance what your maximum pulse rate should be. You can do this by using a simple system of subtraction. Start with 220 and deduct your age. As an example, for a 30-year-old the equation would be as follows:

$$220 - 30 = 190$$

So 190 beats per minute would be their Maximum Training Heart Rate (MTHR). In other words, this is the maximum speed their heart can beat at, so we will call this 100%:

$$220 - 30 = 190 = 100\%.$$

Obviously you don't want to work at 100%. Research has shown that working at approximately 65% is when we burn most fat. 65% of 190 is 123. Therefore, if a 30-year-old reaches a level where their heart is beating 123 times per minute, they are likely to be in their 'fat burning zone'.

$$220 - 30 = 190. \ 65\% \text{ of } 190 = 123.$$

Isn't that good news! Instead of going flat out on an exercise bike or a 'stair climber' and feeling exhausted after five minutes, what you need to do is to pedal away at a level that is comfortable and sustainable. Remember, it takes longer to start burning fat than just glycogen alone, so start gently and gradually increase the time you spend on the activity, until you can work at a comfortable level for 20 or 30 minutes. Rest assured, you *will* be burning fat. You will also be improving your cardiovascular system and reducing your risk of heart disease.

The second school of thought is completely different, but also correct. It is based on the total amount of calories burnt during exercise. Having established that you burn a higher percentage of calories from fat if the level is low to moderate, we now need to look at the total number of calories burnt overall during low versus high intensity exercise. The following table shows the difference between the total calories burnt during walking and running:

	Walking	*Running*
Distance	4 miles/	6 miles/
	6 kilometres	10 kilometres
Speed	4 mph/6 kph	6 mph/10 kph
Time	60 minutes	60 minutes

Total Calories	270	680
% Fat Calories	60	40
Total Fat		
Calories	160	270

By looking at these figures, we can see that we *do* burn a higher percentage of fat calories when the activity is low to moderate, and that it is good news for those of us who don't like to work too hard. However, we must also look at the *total number of fat calories burnt* in order to see the whole picture. Although we burn 60 per cent of calories from fat when we are walking, as opposed to only 40 per cent when running, the total number of fat calories burnt is higher when running, because the overall total is so much greater (40 per cent of 680 is more than 60 per cent of 270). This should not be taken too literally, however, as the figures shown are based on running for 60 minutes, which is unachievable for most of us. I certainly could not run for 60 minutes! These figures are also assuming that the runner can not only run for 60 minutes, but can also remain within their aerobic training zone whilst doing so, continuing to burn fat. This is unrealistic for most people.

For every individual there is a particular point at which we can no longer continue to work aerobically – that is, supply oxygen at the rate it is required. At this point we then start to use the anaerobic energy system (without oxygen), which does not burn fat and in turn produces lactic acid in the muscle. This causes muscle soreness, which eventually stops the muscles from contracting. Whether or not you should walk or jog to burn more fat, therefore, depends largely on your fitness level and on how long you are able to exercise for.

When we compare walking and running over 20 minutes instead of 60, we can see that the difference between total calories burnt and the percentage of fat calories burnt is not so great:

	Walking	Running
Time	20 minutes	20 minutes
Total calories	90	226
% Fat calories	60	40
Total fat calories	54	90

A difference of 36 calories is negligible, especially when you consider that the calories you burn up after exercise are the most significant. Any exercise that you can sustain for 20 minutes or more will increase your metabolic rate for several hours afterwards. If jogging is suitable for you, great; if not, no problem – just walk or do whatever you can.

In addition to this, you should remember that the total amount of calories burnt will vary from one individual to another, according to their total body weight and the amount of Lean Body Mass (*see* page 43). One 1lb/0.4kg of muscle will require approximately 40 calories per day in order to function – excluding exercise. The more you exercise, the more calories the muscle will require – not just when you are exercising but throughout the day and night, as it repairs itself and starts to grow stronger. The result is a higher percentage of muscle on our bodies, so we burn more calories when we work out. This in turn means we burn more calories throughout the day and night, and so the cycle goes on. All these extra calories have to come from somewhere and, providing you are not eating more than you need, they will come from the body's fat stores – the perfect way to lose weight.

EVERYDAY EXERCISE

It is important not to get too 'bogged down' with worrying about which exercise burns the most fat while you are working out. It is the total number of calories you burn in just staying alive that will influence how much or how little fat you burn. Only a small percentage of the calories you burn come from exercise, compared to the amount burnt just keeping you alive.

The exercise programmes set out in this book include both aerobic and anaerobic exercises, in order to stimulate the fat cells into releasing more fat (*see* Chapter 4), to replace muscle tissue and to increase the total amount of fat calories burnt throughout the day – and night. What is vital, however, is that you adapt the programme to suit *you*. For example, when choosing your aerobic activity, it is important to find something that you both *like* to do and are *able* to do for at least 20 minutes – more if possible. You may find that power walking is a comfortable yet challenging work-out for you, if walking at a normal pace is not enough and running is too much. When power walking, you need to take much longer strides and to use your arms and upper body to help you with the momentum. You should use as many of your muscles as possible and not just your legs.

Your body does not know the difference between providing energy for hoovering and providing energy for an aerobics class. When the muscles start to work, the brain receives messages telling it to increase the supply of oxygen. This is the responsibility of the heart, which then has to pump faster to meet the increased demands. Here is a list of every-day activities that you probably do regularly, to show you that you really are burning up calories all day long:

Activity	Calories Per Minute
Driving a car	2.8
Making beds	3.4
Cleaning windows	3.7
Sweeping floors	3.9
Ironing	4.2
Raking the lawn	4.7
Weeding the garden	5.6
Walking upstairs	10.0 or more

You can, therefore, make a considerable difference to the amount of calories you burn simply by being more active in everyday life.

Chapter 6

Perfecting Proportions

Designing Your Exercise Programme

In order to maximize the amount of fat you burn from your body and to make sure that it stays off, you must include both aerobic and strength work.

As you start to exercise more regularly, you will see your shape changing and you will also have more energy. How quickly you start to see and feel these benefits will depend on several factors. *Firstly*, how hard you work. The improvements will occur in direct proportion to the level of overload (challenge) that you place on your body's systems. Complete beginners will achieve benefits from almost any level of exercise – even a gentle walk may be enough to cause the body to change. *Secondly*, how often you exercise. You will need to commit yourself to regular times during the week; the more you do, the quicker you will improve – within reason! *Thirdly*, how long you spend exercising. If you want an aerobic work-out, you should allow 30 minutes or more as you will need to warm up, stretch and cool down. The toning exercises, however, can be done in 15 minutes or less.

We can put these three factors into practice by using a FIT check list:

> **Frequency** = how often?
> **Intensity** = how hard?
> **Time** = how long?

At the end of each week you must check your FIT list to make sure that you have achieved your targets. Fill in the chart as you design your own exercise regime, so that you set aside time in advance to exercise. If you wait for a spare half hour to come along, it never will – you have to *make* time!

	Aerobic	Toning	Combination
Frequency	Monday & Thursday	Wednesday & Friday	Saturday
Intensity	65%		65–75%
Time	30 minutes	15 minutes	60 minutes

By using the chart you can timetable your exercise sessions and see in advance exactly what commitment you need to give to your programme. It is vital that you write it down. If something is in your head, it is a dream, a wish or a hope; once it is written down, it becomes a commitment towards achieving your goal. Get your diary out *now* and timetable your workouts for this week. Make sure you do this at the start of every week.

THE AEROBIC WORK-OUT

In order to work aerobically, your heart needs to be pumping blood and oxygen around your body at the same rate as it is being used. In simple terms, this means that you should be slightly breathless but not gasping. It is impossible to set a level of exercise that is going to be the same for everyone, so you will need to estimate how hard you are working. As mentioned previously, this can be done by taking your age and working out your MTHR (Maximum Training Heart Rate) by deducting your age from 220 (*see* page 104). An easier method is to use a Perceived Rate Of Exertion Scale (PRE Scale), which gives you guidelines as to how you should be feeling. I have devised a simplified version of the PRE Scale, which is much easier to follow :

Level 1   No effort
Level 2   Slight effort
Level 3   Effort required
Level 4   Rate of breathing starts to increase
Level 5   Slightly breathless – starting to perspire
Level 6   Breathless but comfortable – perspiring
             freely

Level 7   More breathless – still able to speak short sentences

Level 8   More breathless – only able to speak a few words

Level 9   Very breathless – unable to speak – feeling tired

Level 10   Very breathless – heavy legs – unable to continue

You should always begin with a warming-up period before you start the activity itself. This should include smaller movements using the same muscles that are going to be challenged when you are working out. For example, walking is a good warm-up exercise if you are going to power walk or jog. You should also include stretches for the leg muscles, as shown on pages 131–135. By the end of the warm up you should be feeling about level 4; you are now ready to begin your aerobic work-out and you should time it from this point. As you start to work a little harder, you should reach approximately level 6 or 7. This will ensure that you are well within your aerobic training zone and that you are burning fat. You should continue to exercise at this level for as long as is comfortable.

THE BENEFITS

The centre of aerobic exercise is the heart, but it also involves many other important organs and systems. Any body system that is challenged will start to improve in efficiency. Aerobic exercise will, therefore, improve the efficiency of the heart, the respiratory system and the muscles used, as well as increasing the metabolism. When aerobic fitness improves, there is a real sense of wellbeing and an enhancement of mental health.

The *heart* is a muscle and, like any other muscle, it can grow stronger and, therefore, do more work with less effort. Imagine a weightlifter picking up a weight that they can lift several times. Compare that to someone who doesn't exercise and who probably is unable to pick it up at all. The weightlifter has stronger muscles – we can train our heart in the same way. The way in which we train aerobically differs from how we strengthen other muscles in our body. We do not want to be able to occasionally do something really strenuous with our heart for a short period of time; we want it to get stronger so that it can carry on beating for longer. This form of training is called 'endurance' training.

One of the ways in which our heart adapts to endurance training is that it increases slightly in size, which means it can pump more blood with every heartbeat – this is called stroke volume. Imagine two sponges: one small, face sponge and one large, bath sponge. If you had a leak or a puddle of water in a cupboard and used the two sponges to soak it up, you would, of course, see a marked difference between the efficiency of the two. The small sponge would fill up quickly and, when you squeezed it out, not much water would pass through it. You would be soaking and wringing it out very quickly, to try to get rid of the water. On the other hand, if you used the big sponge, it would soak up more water so that when you squeezed it out you would be able to pass a lot more water through it. The overall rate would be slower, however, as it would take more time to fill up and to empty. In other words, it would be pumping more slowly, *but* it would clear the water up more quickly and with less effort. It is logical to calculate that the small sponge will wear out very quickly due to overuse, while the life span of the big sponge will be much longer. As your heart increases in size and stroke volume, it will be doing more work with less effort. All your muscles will receive a healthy supply of oxygen and you will literally feel fitter.

Circulation is the process by which the blood is delivered to the muscles and into the cells, using a network of blood vessels. These blood vessels get gradually smaller and smaller until they become tiny capillaries. At this point, the oxygen literally hops off into the cells and carbon dioxide – a waste product of aerobic energy production – hops on and is carried, via the heart, back to the lungs, where it can now be expelled when we breathe out. As we improve the efficiency of our heart, we also improve the efficiency of the capillary network. This means that there are more capillaries passing oxygen into the cells. With all this going on, it is hardly surprising that we start to feel more energetic!

There is no doubt that aerobic exercise is the best way to strengthen your heart and to reduce the risk of heart disease and many other associated diseases. The good news is that *anyone* can do it.

Aerobic exercise adds years to your life and life to your years.

CHOOSE YOUR EXERCISE

Because of the obvious limitations of exercising from a book, I am going to suggest that you choose your aerobic exercise from the following list. Choose two aerobic activities and do these twice per week. Make sure you use your exercise chart to timetable them so that you don't keep putting it off. Think of your exercise sessions as appointments that you *must* keep.

Power Walking

This involves both taking longer strides than you do when you walk normally and moving your arms as well as your legs, so that you can build up some momentum.

Jogging

Do this at a comfortable level that you can maintain. If you start to get breathless and unable to speak, reduce to a power walk. Make sure you wear some good running shoes, particularly if you are running on a concrete surface.

Swimming

When swimming, make sure that you use your legs as well as your arms. Try keeping your arms by your side and just using your legs for some of the time. It doesn't really matter which stroke you use; choose the most comfortable for you, or better still, vary it every few lengths.

Cycling

Cycle at a comfortable level and try to choose a route which you can manage without stopping. Make sure you know what is around the corner. It may feel great going down a hill, but don't forget that you will have to get up the other side! A safety helmet should always be worn, and make sure that your bike is in good working order before you leave.

The Stationary Bike
This is one of the few work-outs where it is possible to take your pulse rate fairly accurately. Pedal for at least five minutes, until you can feel you are perspiring and slightly breathless. Now take your pulse to see how hard you are working, using the MTHR scale (*see* page 104). If you get bored, try putting the bike in front of the television and watching a video or a favourite programme.

Step Machines
These are a relatively new, but very valuable, addition to home exercise equipment. As with the stationary bike, you can place them in front of the television, or exercise while listening to the radio. They are available with a frame to hold on to, or you can also get a smaller version which just has the foot pads. If possible, go for the larger variety, as the range of leg movements is greater. If not, make sure you try to use your arms as well.

The Step
This is a bench for stepping up and down. Always choose a step that has adjustable heights, as you may need to start out at 4 or 6 inches/10 or 15 centimetres, as opposed to the maximum height of 8 inches/20

centimetres. Most steps come with an instructional video – if your step doesn't, you should buy one in order to ensure you are using a good technique. Although the step has been associated with knee injuries, in almost all cases it was because of incorrect step technique. Practised properly, itis an excellent form of cardiovascular exercise. You could also join a step class, but make sure that the instructor teaches you properly (*see* notes on page 93).

Rowing Machines

These can be used for an excellent overall work-out using lots of muscles. Recent studies have shown using a rowing machine to be one of the best forms of exercise for preventing osteoporosis (brittle bones), as it challenges muscles and puts stress on the bones, stimulating healthy bone-cell production.

Aerobics Classes

Exercising in a group setting can often be more motivating. Do make sure, however, that the class you choose is at the appropriate level for you. Don't start off with the advanced class or one that is too heavily choreographed or you will not enjoy it. Make sure the aerobics section of the class lasts at least 20 minutes before going onto toning work. If toning work is included in the class, it will be a good combination work-out.

You can vary your aerobic work-out regularly. If you haven't exercised for a while, try different things until you find something that you enjoy. It doesn't matter what you do as long as you do something! Remember, your heart doesn't know the difference between step and rowing, it just knows that it needs to work harder to pump more oxygen to the muscles. So the more muscles you are using, the better. Use the PRE Scale to monitor how you are feeling. To stay within your aerobic threshold you should not go above level 7.

TONING EXERCISES
(MUSCLE FITNESS)

Toning exercises are often referred to as 'strength work'. Unfortunately, this puts many people off, as they associate strength with heavy weights and bulky muscles. This is not the case, however. It is possible to have a strength work-out just using your body as resistance. This means altering your position in order to make the exercise harder or easier. As with all aspects of fitness, we tend to think of extremes, so visions of Olympic weightlifters spring to mind when we use the word strength. Of course, these athletes do have to lift heavy weights and to train very hard to achieve their desired end result – but our desired result is quite different. We just want to strengthen our muscles so that they can support the weight of our skeleton and frame, to allow us to move and to accomplish everyday tasks more easily. The weightlifter ultimately has to lift a weight, so that is what he trains with. We, on the other hand, only need to lift our body or relatively light weights, so that's what we train with.

THE BENEFITS

As explained in the section on body composition (*see* pages 45–8), we lose muscle naturally as we get older. It literally wastes away, making us weaker. This is a natural process of ageing and we cannot halt it completely. We can, however, drastically reduce the rate at which it takes place, simply by using the muscles more. How sad it would be to reach retirement and not have the physical ability to enjoy the long-awaited fruits of years of hard work. Strength reaches a peak during our early 20s and then starts to decline. With exercise, however, it hardly declines at all. Muscular strength is equally as important to overall health as aerobic fitness – just in a different way.

Complaints of *back pain* seem to have reached epidemic proportions. Numerous surveys have shown that an enormous number of people suffer from back pain at some point in their life, and that weak muscles are most commonly to blame. There is a balance between the front and the back of the body, which must be maintained in order to ensure correct posture. Strong abdominal muscles are very important to ensure stability of the spine. We should also work the muscles in the back, so that together the two muscle groups can hold us upright and allow the spine to move without suffering from stress.

Think of the spine as a pile of dominoes, balanced one on top of the other. If you change the position of one near the bottom of the pile, it will affect the stability of the dominoes at the top. For the pile to remain stable, it is also important to balance them all correctly. Our spine is set in a delicate alignment, and, unlike the dominoes, it is 'S' shaped. This is so that it can withstand maximum stress and impact. Any forces that strike at the feet are passed up the spine and need to be dissipated or reduced, to prevent the vibrations from reaching the brain. This is why correct technique and appropriate footwear are so important when running. If you are heavy footed, as your foot strikes the ground, the shock it has to pass on is much greater and, therefore, the risk of injury much higher.

Osteoporosis is becoming more common as more people are living longer. Until recently, it was thought of as a natural process of ageing and believed to be both unavoidable and untreatable. Thankfully, we now know much more about it and more research is currently underway. What we have learnt already is that it is totally preventable and that exercise is the key. When we contract a muscle, it pulls on a bone causing movement. For example, if you bend your elbow, your biceps muscle literally pulls the bones in your lower arm closer to the bones in your upper arm. As it does this, it puts stress on the bone where it is attached – rather like a tug of war team, where the anchor man withstands maximum stress from the pull of the rope. Because he doesn't want to move, he digs his heels in to provide a more stable base. The pull of a muscle on a bone means that the bone needs to withstand the stress of that pulling force, so it produces a higher rate of bone growth, in order to prevent any weakening. Controlled strength exercises, such as those shown in this book, can put enough stress on the bone to stimulate improvements and reduce our risk of suffering from this terrible debilitating disease.

Men and women have a different potential for *building strength*. Men are naturally more muscular due to a hormone called testosterone. The presence of this hormone also means that if they do strength work, they will increase the size of their muscles. Women, on the other hand, don't have the same potential to build muscle bulk. Many women are, however, put off strength training because of a fear of developing 'big muscles'. This fear is unfounded.

Some female body builders have only achieved big muscles by taking testosterone supplements or similar substances and by using very heavy weights. They often develop other characteristics such as a deep voice as well! So if you are worried about building big muscles, don't be – the exercises devised in this book are designed to improve muscle tone and not muscle size, and there is no testosterone included in the diet! The only muscle tissue you will be building will be to replace the muscle tissue that you have been losing for years.

So many things we do every day require strength. In a typical day off, for example, I will usually do the following: take my three children to school; do some housework (moving chairs and other furniture to hoover behind them); carry baskets of laundry upstairs and downstairs; and venture around the supermarket. Shopping for a family of five, two dogs and a cat is enough to fill any trolley to the brim! I use almost all of my muscles trying to steer the trolley through the aisles without crashing into anyone, and then, of course, it needs to be loaded into the car, unloaded the other end and put away. Next it's time to pick the children up and walk the dogs, throwing sticks and balls across a field for the dogs, before going home to cook the dinner. When I actually take time to analyse my activities throughout the day, I am using my muscles all the time – so they need to be strong.

On a typical working day, I am on the go all the time. At the health and fitness club I teach fitness classes and help people around the gym all day, so the amount of calories I can burn in one day is very high for someone of my size. I have to make sure that I eat well so that I have enough energy for my muscles to do all this work, and I must also make sure that the exercise programme I do myself is well balanced so that my posture is good and I am less likely to suffer an injury.

The main advantage of strength training to promote weight-loss, as explained several times in this book, is that the increase in muscle tissue and tone (Lean Body Mass) means that we will burn more calories all day – not just when we are exercising. Take the list of things that I might do in a day off, for example. Because my ratio of LBM is good since I exercise regularly, I am burning more calories even when I do the shopping. My posture is good and I have drastically reduced my risk of suffering from osteoporosis. By following the exercise programmes in this book, you can achieve all these things for yourself.

HOW HARD YOU WORK

You want to strengthen your muscles to help you in everyday life, so you don't need to lift heavy weights and to go through pain. With aerobic exercises you should always feel comfortable and able to do more; with strength exercises you should feel really challenged by the end of each 'set'. When you do the exercises, although I have suggested the amount of repetitions you should do, you may need to vary this to suit your own ability. If you are doing ten repetitions of something and then stopping, that represents one set. At the end of the set, if you feel as if you could have done a few more, then you have not worked hard enough. If you don't really challenge the muscle it won't improve. If ten is the absolute maximum you can do and the last one is painful, then you are working too hard and should stop at eight or nine.

There is a difference between fatigue and failure; fatigue means that the muscle feels tired after you have completed the set and that you feel you have really achieved something. This is the level you want to aim for. Failure means that the last exercise (repetition) in the set was painful and that you couldn't complete it properly. You should avoid this stage as your muscles are likely to be very sore a day or two later and you may injure yourself. It is very important when doing strength work that you work to fatigue *not* failure.

The toning exercises I have devised can easily be done at home. They should take approximately 15 minutes or less, including some warm-up and stretching exercises. There are two programmes, although some of the exercises are the same in both. The programmes have been carefully designed to balance muscle strength evenly to promote good posture.

THE COMBINATION WORK-OUT

I have included a combination work-out which you should do at least once per week. A combination work-out is a programme including both aerobic and muscular strength work to promote overall fitness. Simply choose one of the aerobic exercises suggested and one of the toning work-outs. For example, you could start with a warm-up followed by 20 minutes or more of power walking, and then come home to do the toning exercises, followed by a good stretch. I suggest you allow an hour for this, although you may find you can do it in less.

The exercise programme I have given you – aerobics twice per week, strength twice per week and one combination work-out – is enough for you to really see and feel the benefits. If you practise this programme conscientiously and follow the diet, you *will* succeed. If you choose to exercise more frequently that is fine, but make sure you have one day per week when you do no exercise, in order to allow the body to rest and recover. Exercise is clearly a good thing. If you go over sensible limits, however, it can be a bad thing, and you may end up feeling run down and unwell. I hope you have learnt from reading this book that losing weight should not mean going through torture sessions, and that you can achieve really good results without breaking the pain barrier!

Once you have achieved your goal, you will need to exercise regularly to maintain it, although you can reduce the frequency to two or three times per week. I recommend one toning work-out, one aerobic and one combination.

WARMING UP

Before commencing any kind of work-out, you should always begin with a warm-up. This is essential because it reduces the risk of injury, which can be quite high if the body is not prepared properly. The type of warm-up exercise you should do depends on the kind of exercises you will be doing in your work-out.

THE AEROBIC WARM-UP

The purpose of the aerobic warm-up is to raise the pulse to a comfortable level so that you can exercise safely within your 'training zone'. For example, if you are power walking, you should begin by walking at a normal pace and circle your shoulders slowly until you feel your heart rate has increased and you have reached level 4 on the PRE Scale (*see* pages 113–14). The principle is the same for all the aerobic activities – that is, start swimming, cycling, stepping or rowing at a gentle pace and then gradually increase it. When you feel your pulse rate has achieved level four (PRE Scale), you should then do the following stretches:

Front of Thigh (Quads)

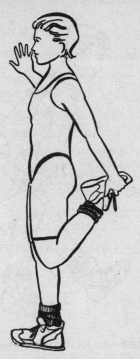

Using a wall for balance, place one foot in your hand and ease the leg back slowly until the knee is behind the hip. Keep the hips square, pull your tummy in to support your back and tilt your pelvis under. You should feel the stretch across the front of the hip and down the front of the thigh. Hold for eight – ten seconds, then repeat with the other leg.

Back of Thigh (Hamstrings)

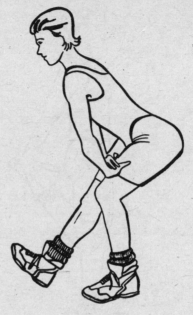

Stand with one foot in front of the other, as if you had taken a generous stride forwards, and transfer all of your weight to your back leg; bending the leg, sit down into the stretch. Support your body weight with both hands on the thigh of the bent leg, and tilt the pelvis so that the base of your spine is inclined towards the ceiling. Keep the hips square. You should feel this down the back of the straight leg, from the hip to just below the knee. Hold for eight–ten seconds, then repeat with the other leg.

Calf (Gastrocnemius)

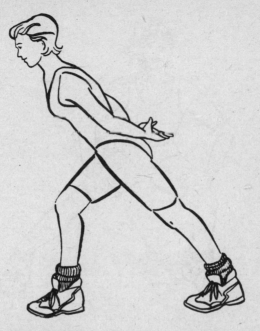

Stand with one foot in front of the other, as if you had taken a generous stride ahead. Bend the front leg and transfer the body weight forwards; make sure that the heel of the back foot is on the floor and that the toes are facing forwards. Press the hips forwards to ensure that a diagonal line runs down the body from your head to your toes. Hold for eight–ten seconds, then repeat with the other leg.

Inner Thigh (Adductors)

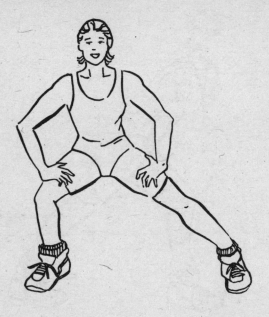

Stand with your feet wide apart. Bend one leg and transfer the body weight over to this leg. Make sure that your knee does not go over the line of your toe. You should be able to see your foot – if not, your feet are too close together. Keep the hips square to the front. You should feel this on the inside thigh of the straight leg. Hold for eight–ten seconds, and repeat with the other leg.

Outer Thigh (Abductors)

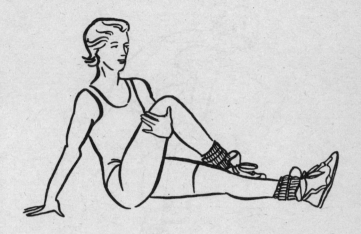

Sit on the floor with the left leg straight in front of you. Bend the right knee and cross it over the left leg, keep the right hand on the floor and, using the left hand, pull the right knee gently towards you. You should feel the stretch in the outside of the right thigh. Hold for eight–ten seconds, and repeat with the other leg.

Back (Erector Spinae)

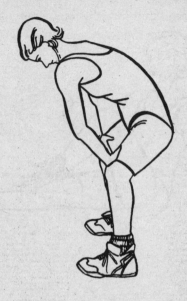

Stand with your feet slightly wider apart than hip width, bend the knees and lower into a squatting position. Place your hands just above your knees and support your body weight in your arms. Pull the tummy in, and tuck your head and pelvis under to arch the spine. You should feel this all the way down the back. Hold for eight–ten seconds, then repeat.

THE TONING WARM-UP

It is not necessary to raise the pulse for toning work, but you should mobilize the joints that you are going to use. Repeat the following exercises eight–ten times.

Shoulder Circles

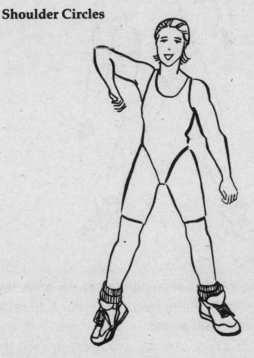

Stand with the feet apart and transfer the weight from side to side. As you do this, circle alternate shoulders. Start with small circles and increase the size of the circles gradually until you are doing full-arm circles.

Side Bends

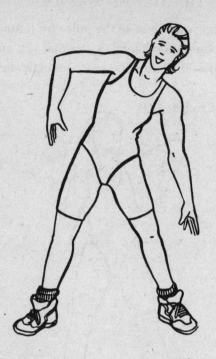

Stand with your feet hip-width apart. Keeping the hips square to the front, lean slowly down to each side, as far as is comfortable.

Knee Lifts

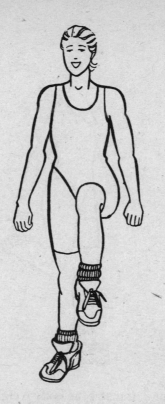

Raise alternate knees to hip height, pulling the tummy in as you lift, to support the back.

Hamstring Curls

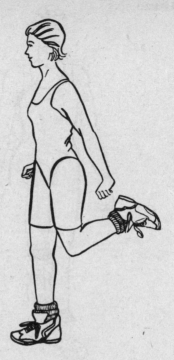

With feet apart, transfer the body weight from one leg to the other. Kick back with alternate legs so that your heel comes towards your bottom.

After you have done the mobility exercises above, you will need to do the stretches shown for the aerobic warm-up. In addition to these, you should also stretch some other muscles that you will be using during the toning section by doing the following exercises.

Chest (Pectorals)

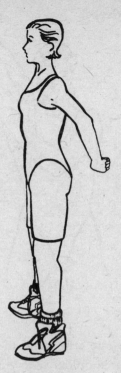

Stand with the feet apart and place your hands on your bottom. Gently squeeze your elbows together behind your back. You should feel the stretch across the front of the chest and the shoulders. Hold for eight–ten seconds.

Upper Arm (Triceps)

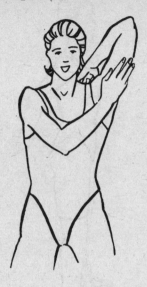

Reach up with one arm, bend the elbow and touch the back of your shoulder with your hand. Using the other arm, gently push the arm back. You should feel the stretch down the back of the arm. Hold for eight–ten seconds.

Upper Back (Trapezius and Rhomboids)

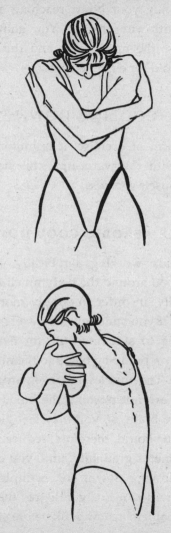

Stand with your feet apart. Fold your arms in front of you and hug your body, reaching around your shoulders with your hands. You should feel the stretch across the upper back and the back of the shoulders. Hold for eight–ten seconds.

COOLING DOWN

After any form of exercise, it is important to cool down. As with the warm-ups, this helps prevent injury and muscle soreness.

THE AEROBIC COOL DOWN

When you are working aerobically, the heart is pumping blood around the body much faster than it does normally, in order to supply more oxygen to the muscles. If you suddenly stop exercising – going from running to standing still, for example – the heart carries on pumping blood to the muscles at this elevated rate. The muscles, however, are not contracting, so they are not pushing the blood back to the heart and the brain, so you may feel giddy or even pass out. You should, therefore, reduce the intensity of the movements gradually, until you can feel your heart rate slowing down. For example, if you are running, slow down to a gentle jog, then to a brisk walk, and finally to a slow walk before stopping. The amount of time it takes to cool down depends on your fitness level. Initially it may take four–five minutes, but as your body becomes used to exercise you will be able to reduce your pulse rate in two–three minutes.

Another reason for cooling down is to give the muscles the chance to flush out any lactic acid. Just as you flush the chain on the toilet, the 'new' blood is flushed into the muscle forcing the 'used' blood out. The waste products – that is, lactic acid – are then carried back to the liver where they are broken down and disposed of. If you have ever experienced muscle soreness after a work-out, it is more likely to be because you did not cool down properly than because you were working too hard, although working too hard can also cause pain and soreness a day or too after exercise.

COOL-DOWN STRETCHES

After any kind of work-out you should stretch the muscles you have been using, to prevent muscle stiff-ness and promote flexibility. Repeat the stretches you did before the work-out.

TONING PROGRAMME 1

Front of Thigh (Quads)

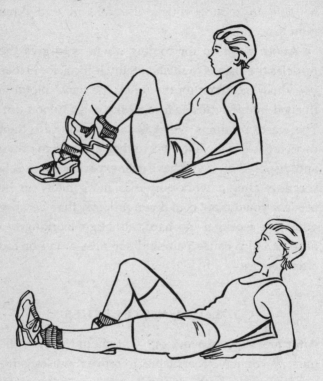

From sitting up, lean back so that you are supporting your weight on your elbows, keep your tummy pulled in tightly to support your back, and bend one knee so that your foot is close to your bottom. Bend

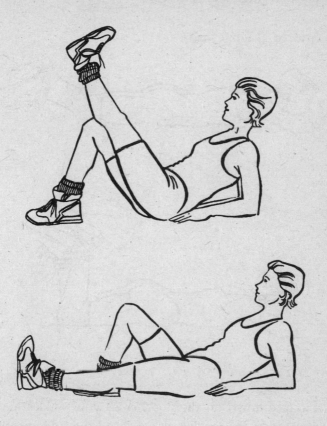

the other leg in towards your chest, extend it keeping
it just off the floor and then lift and lower it carefully.
Repeat the whole movement.

Suggested repetitions: 10/12 each leg

Back of Thigh (Hamstrings)

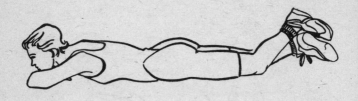

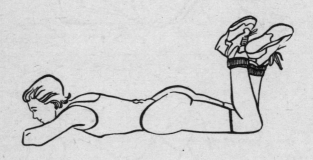

Lie face down on the floor, cross your ankles and resist with the top leg as you bend the underneath leg. You can add as much or as little pressure as is comfortable.

Suggested repetitions: 8/10 each leg

Outer Thigh (Abductors)

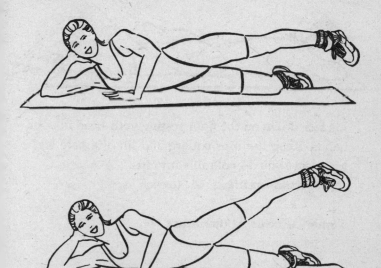

Lie on your side supporting your neck in your hand. Bend the underneath leg and straighten the top leg. Make sure that your hips are square to the front, then raise and lower the top leg, leading with the heel. Aim to touch the toe on the floor each time you lower your leg.

Suggested repetitions: 10/12 each leg

Bottom (Gluteuls)

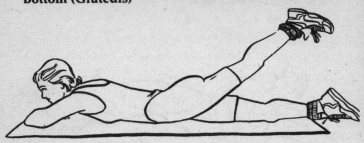

Lie face down on the floor resting your head in your hands. Keep the hips square and lift alternate legs. Make sure you do not roll your hips.

Suggested repetitions: 14/16 each leg

Tummy (Rectus Abdominus)

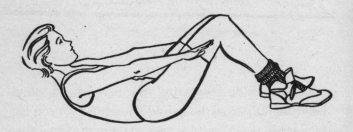

Lie on your back with your knees bent. Press your tummy down into the floor and, as you do so, curl your ribs towards your hips, then lower down and

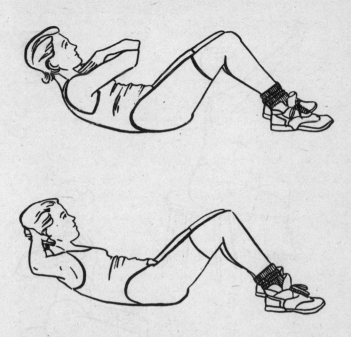

repeat. Think of it as a curling movement and not a lift. You can select a hand position that is most comfortable for you, either across the chest or beside the head to make it more difficult. You may need to support your neck by placing your hand on the back of your neck and allowing your head to rest on your forearm as you curl up.

Suggested repetitions: 10/12

Upper Back (Trapezius & Rhomboids)

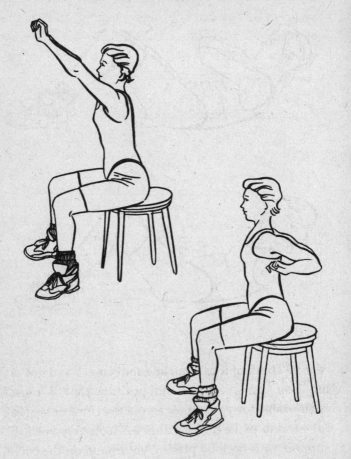

Sit upright on a chair, close to the front. Reach upwards and forwards. Pull your arms back and down in a diagonal line, trying to squeeze your shoulder blades together as you do so. Reach up and repeat. You can hold light weights, such as tins of food, to make this more difficult as you grow stronger.

Suggested repetitions: 10/12

Upper Arm (Biceps)

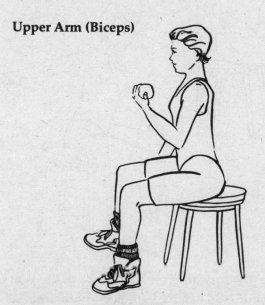

Sitting upright on a chair, hold a light weight in each hand – a tin of food, for example. Raise your arms slightly in front of you and bend each arm alternately. Keep your elbows close to your body.

Suggested repetitions: 16/18 each arm

Back of Arm (Triceps)

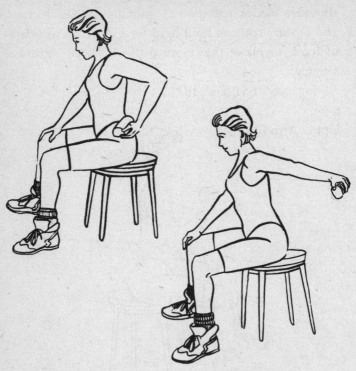

Sitting slightly forwards on the chair, place your hands by your side behind you. Bend both arms so that your hands are hip height and your elbows are well behind you. Keeping the top of your arm still, straighten one elbow, then bend it back to the original position and repeat with the other arm. Keep your tummy pulled in to support your back.

Suggested repetitions: 12/14 each arm

TONING PROGRAMME 2

Legs (Quads, Gluteuls and Hamstrings)

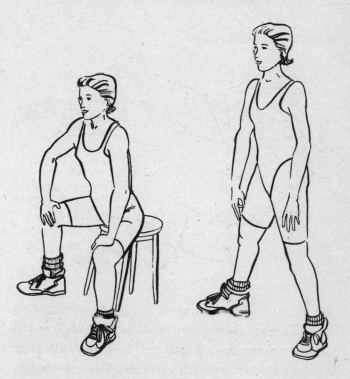

Sit on a chair with your feet slightly apart. Place your hands on your thighs and stand up. As you do so, press your hips forwards. From the standing position, bend the knees and slowly lower yourself back down into a sitting position. As you get stronger, you can do this without the chair, but make sure that your bottom doesn't go below your knees as you squat down.

Suggested repetitions: 10/12

Inner Thigh (Adductors)

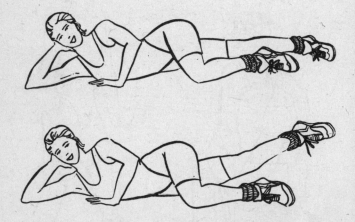

Lie on your side with your top leg bent across so that your knee is level with your hips. Straighten the underneath leg so that your heel is in line with your hips, not in front or behind. Keeping this leg straight, lift it as high as possible *without* turning the hips, and then lower it without putting the weight back onto the floor. After you have finished the whole set, repeat using the other leg.

Suggested repetitions: 8/10

Tummy (Rectus Abdominus)

Follow the instructions on pages 150–51.

Chest (Pectorals)

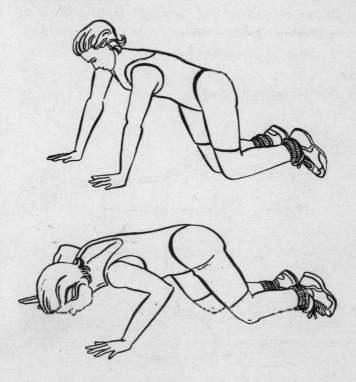

On your hands and knees, place your hands slightly wider than your shoulders and make sure that your chin is in line with your fingers. Pull your tummy in to support your back, and bend your arms slowly, lowering your nose almost to the floor. Straighten your arms and push back up again.

If this is too difficult for you, or is painful for your wrists, lie on your back on the floor with your arms bent (hold cans of food to make it more challenging) and bring your forearms together. Lower and repeat.

Suggested repetitions: 6/8

Back (Erector Spinae)

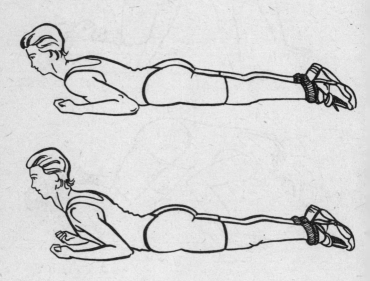

Lie on your front with your arms bent close to your body, placing your hands slightly wider than your shoulders with palms turned up. Using the muscles

in your back, raise your shoulders slightly off the
floor. Your elbows will provide stability but should
not do the work. Lower slowly and repeat.

Suggested repetitions: 6/8

Waist (Obliques)

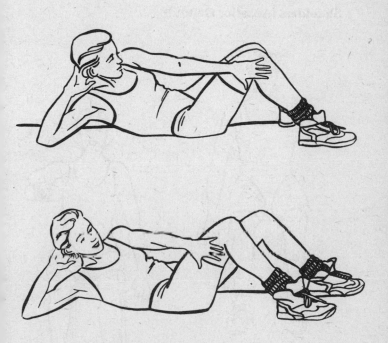

Lie on your back with your knees bent and your feet
slightly apart. Keeping the hips still, lift and turn your
upper body so that you touch the outside of the

opposite thigh with your hand. You may need to support the neck with the other hand as you do this. You must aim to curl the ribs towards the hips and turn at the same time, without rolling the hips. Lower slowly and carefully and repeat.

Suggested repetitions: 8 each side

Shoulders (Anterior Deltoid)

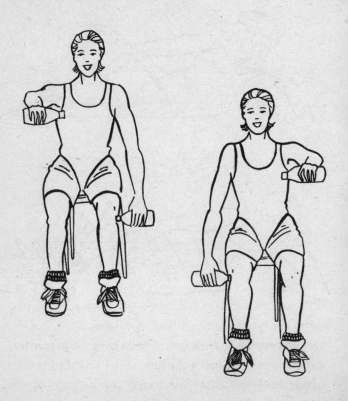

Sitting on a chair, holding a light weight in each hand (a tin of food, for example), pull your tummy in to support your back. Raise alternate arms in front of you to just above shoulder height. Lower slowly.

Suggested repetitions: 12/14 each arm

Shoulders (Superior Deltoid)

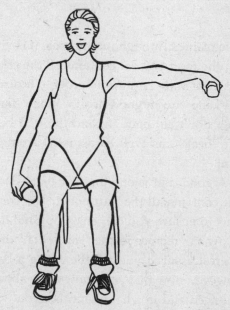

Sitting on a chair as before, raise alternate arms to the side. Keep your hands in line with your body, not in front or behind. Lift each arm to just above shoulder height and lower slowly.

Suggested repetitions: 12/14 each arm

Chapter 7

The 'Fat to Flat' Diet

28 Days – The Recipes for Success

As explained throughout the book, it is vital to ensure that the food you eat contains all the essential nutrients your body requires in order to function properly and keep you in good health. When dieting, people often don't eat enough, and this can be harmful to your health, as well as actually promoting weight gain!

A good diet is one that is balanced – that is, one that contains all the nutrients in the correct proportions to ensure you can enjoy optimal health. If you follow the recipes in the 'Fat to Flat' diet, then you can rest assured you will be eating a balanced diet. However, now that you know more about what food you need and in what quantities, you will be able to plan your own balanced diet providing you stick to the guidelines I have laid out for you.

This 28-day diet plan has been carefully designed to ensure maximum nutritional content *and* maximum taste. So often we associate diets with tasteless and boring meals, such as lettuce leaf sandwiches. In this book, however, you will find the recipes mouth-watering and delicious. My thanks to Sharman Thomson, a cordon-bleu chef, for her expertise in helping me to select the right ingredients and cooking methods to ensure that every meal is delicious.

If you follow this plan you will not only lose weight, but you are also more likely to stay in good health and feel full of vitality.

The plan is easy to follow, and can be adapted to suit different tastes as well as different circumstances. There are, however, a few guidelines which you should follow strictly. These are all outlined below.

BREAKFAST – KICK START THE METABOLISM

Always have breakfast – it is vital to get your metabolism going. Choose something from the following sections.

CEREAL

Most people start the day with cereal, which can be very nutritious. You should, however, avoid the sugar-coated varieties, even if they are promoted as being 'low fat' (some 'low-fat' cereals are actually coated with more sugar than the regular varieties). Always check the label for this before you buy. Beware of refined cereals as well, as these have all undergone a vigorous processing procedure. Although many cereals advertise 'fortified with vitamins and minerals', what this really means is that they have stripped the cereal of all its natural nutritional content in the processing, and only replaced a few known nutrients.

If you are used to sugar-coated cereals and don't like the taste of the bran-type cereals, try weaning yourself off slowly. I was a frosties fan for many years and gradually started to mix in some bran flakes. I started off with a mix of 80 per cent frosties, 20 per cent bran flakes, and worked my way down to bran flakes with some fruit, to replace the sweet taste. Now that I have re-educated my palate, I usually have porridge with bran and some chopped fruit, which sets me up for the day. If you prefer, you can also mix your cereal with low-fat yogurt or low-fat fromage frais instead of milk. This can really enhance the taste of the more bland varieties.

Here are my recommendations for cereals:

- Porridge (preferably organically grown) with water and/or skimmed milk.
- Bran flakes with skimmed milk and a fresh piece of chopped fruit.
- Bran cereal with skimmed milk and a fresh piece of chopped fruit.

- Two wheat biscuits with skimmed milk, sweetened with honey (preferably organically produced) if necessary.
- Muesli with skimmed milk – beware of some brands which contain a large quantity of nuts, as these can be very high in fat. Always check the packet before you buy.

IF YOU DON'T LIKE CEREAL

- Fresh fruit – two pieces of the fruit of your choice, peeled and chopped into small pieces, with low-fat yogurt, fromage frais or skimmed milk. Alternatively, if you are eating breakfast 'on the run', take two pieces of fruit with you to eat on the journey, and a carton of juice (pure with no added sugar).
- Toast – two slices of thickly cut brown bread. Do not spread with butter, have jam or honey instead (organic honey if possible). (Some people feel very 'bloated' and suffer from constipation when they eat bread. This is quite common and can be due to an intolerance of wheat. If this applies to you, you may be able to tolerate white bread only, but if not, avoid bread altogether.)

LIGHT LUNCHES

Always have lunch. If you don't have time to prepare some of the lunches I have included, then select some of the easier alternatives instead, such as a sandwich. This is also more practical if you take a packed lunch to work.

As you will see, I have included several soups on the lunch-time menus, and for one person these will make enough for several days and can be frozen. You can make the soups thicker or thinner, according to preference, simply by using more or less stock. All soups should be served with a large wholemeal roll or a thick slice of wholemeal bread.

Where a sandwich or jacket potato is shown, select one of the fillings listed below (use two or three slices of wholemeal or Granary bread for the sandwich):

- tuna fish (in spring water) and a pinch of fresh basil
- cottage cheese and pineapple
- salmon and cucumber
- salad with a touch (¼ tsp) of horseradish
- cottage cheese with finely chopped celery and apple
- sardines (in tomato juice, not oil) and watercress
- mangetout and tomatoes finely chopped with ¼ tsp of mixed-grain mustard

- humus, cucumber and a pinch of dill
- watercress, grated carrots and cottage cheese
- cottage cheese, a finely chopped peach and ¼ tsp mustard
- tuna (in spring water) with a pinch of coriander
- humus with tomato and black pepper
- mixed bean salad, drained – suitable for jacket potato only
- baked beans – suitable for jacket potato only

HUMUS

I have listed humus above as a sandwich filling. However, many shop-bought varieties are very high in fat (some as much as 85 per cent fat!), so I recommend that you make your own. It's very quick and easy to do – it takes about five minutes and can be kept in the fridge for about four days, or according to the date shown on the yogurt. You can adjust the texture a little by adding more or less yogurt. You will need:

400g/13oz chick peas, blended (with a fork or in a blender) for a smoother texture
150g–200g/5–7oz low-fat fromage frais or plain yogurt
pinch of black pepper and lemon juice, to taste
1 clove garlic, chopped

Mix all the ingredients together in a bowl and place in the fridge to cool.

YOUR EVENING MEAL

Try not to eat your evening meal too late. I have put the largest meal in the evening simply because that is the most common time for people to eat it. However, if it does suit your timetable to eat your main meal at lunch time, that's fine, in fact it's preferable.

The recipes for the main meal serve four people. Obviously this can be halved for two people or you can also freeze some of the meals (this is indicated at the bottom of the relevant recipes). As a working mum, I find it very useful to have some nutritious meals ready in the freezer, as this stops the temptation to get a takeaway after a busy day when you feel too tired to cook!

As with the lunch-time menus, it's not essential that you have everything in the order shown. For example, if you dislike the recipe for a particular day, simply swap that meal for one you prefer from another day. I have included several fish recipes as fish is an excellent source of essential fatty acids (EFAs). Even if you don't normally eat fish, try these recipes – they are delicious. You should eat fish at least once a week.

As you will see, the main meal does not state what you should serve with it as this is up to you. However, you *must* have either a large portion of salad (see below) or at least two vegetables (lightly cooked) with every meal. You should also choose either potatoes, rice (preferably whole-grain) or pasta. It is very important that you feel satisfied after each meal – if you do not, have a low-fat yogurt or a low-fat fromage frais with some chopped fruit in it.

SALAD

I tend to make a large salad every four days and keep it in an airtight container in the fridge. Providing the container is clean and dry when you put the salad in, it will remain fresh. This saves making up a salad every day, which can be time-consuming. You can vary the ingredients in terms of quantities, and according to taste and what is available, but it must include at least some, if not all, of the following:

- lettuce
- raw spinach leaves
- chopped broccoli
- chopped cauliflower
- mangetout
- sprouting beans (fresh)
- chopped or grated carrot
- chopped raw pepper

- sliced courgettes
- 1 level dstsp sesame seeds per salad bowl

FOR VEGETARIANS

I have included a vegetarian option for every meal containing meat. I recommend that you eat the fish dishes as these are essential to ensure an adequate intake of nutrients. If you do not eat fish, simply select one of the other vegetarian options. I would urge you, however, to take professional nutritional advice, as you may need to supplement some nutrients, particularly vitamin B_{12}.

THE DESSERT TROLLEY

As you will see, I have not included a dessert with meals as it is not essential. You should try to educate your palate not to expect something sweet after every meal. However, if you do want to have something simple after your meal, choose a low-fat yogurt, fromage frais or some fresh fruit. Alternatively, if you're planning a special meal, there are a few alternatives listed below. Please remember, however, that just because these desserts are low in fat, it doesn't mean that you can eat twice as much! Give yourself a modest portion and don't have seconds!

Fat-Free Mousse

Serves 2

A delicious and light dessert which will accompany any main meal beautifully. It can be made in any flavour – my personal favourites are pineapple and black cherry.

125g/4oz jelly
200g/7oz fat-free yogurt of the same flavour

1. Melt the jelly according to the instructions on the packet and place in the fridge to cool.
2. When the jelly is semi-set, whisk in the yogurt. Return to the fridge to cool fully before serving.

Rice Pudding

Serves 2–4

1 packet rice pudding
jam or honey (organic if possible)/fresh fruit of your choice

1. Make the rice pudding according to the instructions on the packet using long-life skimmed milk.

2. Sweeten with the jam or honey or chop some
    fruit and stir in as you serve.

Hot Fruit Salad

Serves 4

2 medium-sized bananas
300g/10oz tinned mandarins in fruit juice
2 large oranges, cut into segments
cinnamon, to taste
300g/10oz low-fat fromage frais

1. Place the fruit in a large frying pan or wok, add
    the juice from the mandarins and heat slowly.
2. Add the cinnamon and bring to the boil.
    Continue to boil until the juice has evaporated.
3. Serve immediately with the fromage frais.

Summer Fruit Flan

Serves 4

3 eggs
75g/3oz caster sugar
75g/3oz plain flour
150g/5oz fromage frais
1 small punnet of strawberries and/or raspberries

1. Preheat the oven to 150°C/300°F/gas mark 2.
2. Break the eggs into a bowl and add the sugar.
3. Place the bowl inside a larger bowl containing freshly boiled water and whisk the eggs until *very* stiff. Remove the bowl from the water and continue to whisk until the bowl has completely cooled.
4. Sift the flour and fold into the eggs very carefully, 25g/1oz at a time. Place the mixture in a 15cm/6in non-stick cake tin and bake in the oven for 10–15 minutes.
5. When the sponge has cooled, slice off the top carefully so that the surface is level. Spread the fromage frais onto the surface and decorate with the fruit.

Upside-Down Cheesecake

Serves 6

300g/10oz tinned mandarins or pineapple in juice (preferably not syrup)
1 sachet of gelatine
375g/12oz fromage frais
2 egg whites
8 low-fat digestive biscuits, crushed

1. Drain the fruit and pour the juice into a small jug

or cup. Fill a large bowl with freshly boiled water and place the cup/jug inside the bowl.

2. Allow the gelatine to dissolve in the juice. Remove the cup/jug from the hot water and allow to cool.

3. Fold the drained fruit into the fromage frais and slowly pour in the gelatine/juice mixture.

4. Whisk the egg whites until they are very stiff and then fold them carefully into the mixture. Place this in a loose-bottomed non-stick 20cm/8in tin and put the biscuit crumbs over the top of the cheesecake. (It is not essential to use biscuit crumbs – the cheesecake will be delicious as it is and, of course, lower in fat.)

5. Place in the fridge to cool and set before serving.

SUNDAY ROAST

I have not included a roast dinner in the plan, although the Sunday meals are substantial (if you start the plan on a Monday, they will fall automatically on days 7, 14, 21 and 28). If you would prefer to have a 'traditional' Sunday roast, however, it is not a problem, providing you make a few alterations to the traditional way of cooking it. These are all outlined in the tips below.

The danger with a roast dinner is that we tend to

pile our plates high and eat far more than we actually need. Be sensible when you serve up; don't take any more than you actually need to satisfy you. Stuffing is not recommended, and if you feel you need one, the fat-free mousse shown on page 171 makes an ideal light dessert to accompany your roast dinner.

My tips for cooking a healthy roast:

- Select chicken or turkey, and remove the skin *before* cooking. Place 1 level tsp tarragon and a generous pinch of mixed herbs inside the bird and lay it in a large roasting tin with a lid or foil to cover. Mix a cup of vegetable/chicken stock with hot water and pour into the roasting tin. Place a sheet of greaseproof paper over the bird and put the lid or foil back on to seal. Cook for the recommended time, then leave to stand for 5–10 minutes, keeping the lid on. Remove the meat, drain and carve.

- Peel and parboil the potatoes. Using a pastry brush, paint the bottom of a roasting tin very lightly with extra virgin olive oil and put in the oven to heat. Sprinkle ½–1 tsp dried rosemary over the parboiled potatoes and place in the hot tin. Cook for up to an hour, turning at least once. Alternatively, sprinkle the potatoes with rosemary and then dry-roast them.

- Boil your vegetables – fresh vegetables of your choice and at least one dark green variety – in your usual way and save the water from the cooking for the gravy.

- To make your gravy, take a little of the stock from the chicken/turkey and place in a fat-separating jug. Leave to stand for 5 minutes in a cool place. Using the vegetable water, season to taste with a vegetable or chicken stock cube, add 2 tbsp of the meat stock (once it has separated from the fat) and stir over a low heat. Mix 1–2 tbsp cornflour with some water and stir until it makes a smooth paste. Remove the gravy from the heat and add in the cornflour slowly. Replace over a low heat and continue to stir until the gravy reaches the desired consistency.

FRUIT

When planning your food for the day, you *must* include three pieces of fruit. This is very important as it ensures that you will be getting adequate amounts of fibre and other nutrients. You can either have the fruit as part of a meal – chopped banana in your porridge, for example – or on its own as a snack between meals.

WHAT TO DRINK

Water is undoubtedly the best drink, particularly if you have a water filter. There is a lot of controversy over what and how much you should drink with a meal. Tea and coffee should definitely be avoided within 30 minutes either side of a meal, as they reduce the amount of nourishment you can absorb from your food drastically. Fruit juice is fine, provided that it doesn't have added sugar – always check the packet for details as clever marketing can be misleading. Even pure fruit juice is best diluted.

Drinks to avoid are those in cans, which are packed full of preservatives, sugar or artificial sweeteners – don't be fooled just because it says 'sugar free'. These drinks have absolutely no nutritional value whatsoever and will rot your teeth, not to mention your insides. Other drinks to watch out for are some squashes which are also packed with sugar and preservatives.

So called 'energy drinks' can be made easily and cheaply at home, without any of the additives: dilute some fresh juice of your choice with water – about 30 per cent juice, 70 per cent water – add a pinch of salt and stir well. The only thing contained in these sports drinks that is of value is the salt (electrolytes), which helps to ensure that the body absorbs the fluid quickly. It is the water the body needs most of all in order to keep on performing and not the glucose or sugar.

Throughout the day you should sip water regularly, every time you go into the kitchen at home or the canteen at work. Have a small glass of water even if you are not thirsty. If you are feeling thirsty, then your body is probably already 30 per cent dehydrated!

ALCOHOL

The body cannot use alcohol for muscular work. In other words, it cannot be burnt off, and it also has little or no nutritional value. It makes sense, therefore, not too have too much of it. In this plan I recommend a maximum of one glass of wine or spirit three or four times per week. This does not mean, however, that you can save up your allowance and have it all in one go on a Saturday night! If you do this, your total calories for that day will be excessive and excess calories, no matter what foods they come from, end up as fat.

RECIPES

DAY 1

LUNCH

Pizza Bread

Serves 1

200g/7oz tinned tomatoes
½ small onion, chopped
1 tsp tomato purée
pinch of oregano (optional)
2 medium slices bread
25g/1oz cottage cheese

1. Simmer the tomatoes, onion, purée and oregano for approximately 10 minutes, until they are reduced to a thick purée.
2. Toast the bread on one side. Spread the mixture over the other side and then dot this lightly with the cottage cheese.
3. Grill for 1–2 minutes on a low/moderate heat.

DINNER

Sweet and Sour Pork or Chicken

Serves 4

2 cloves garlic, crushed
¼ tsp chilli powder
25g/1oz fresh root ginger, peeled and chopped
375g/12oz chicken or pork, cut into cubes
½ tsp sesame oil
1 green pepper, diced
1 red pepper, diced
1 large onion, chopped
2 medium carrots, sliced thinly
3 slices of fresh or tinned pineapple, cubed

Sauce

4 tbsp white wine vinegar
2 tbsp cornflour
2 tbsp soy sauce
25g/1oz brown sugar
2 tbsp tomato purée

1. Mix the garlic, chilli and ginger in with the meat, cover and place in the fridge for at least 2 hours.
2. Heat the sesame oil gently in a pan, add the meat and cook for several minutes, stirring

continuously. Remove the meat and place in a dish.

3. Add the vegetables and the pineapple to the pan and stir fry for two minutes. Remove and add to the meat.

4. To make the sauce, add 1–2 tbsp white wine vinegar to the cornflour in a bowl to make a paste. Put the soy sauce, remaining vinegar, sugar and tomato purée into the pan and heat to just boiling. Pour this onto the cornflour mixture and stir until all paste is dissolved.

5. Pour the sauce back into the pan, stirring all the time to make sure it's smooth. Return the meat and vegetables to the pan and cook with the sauce for 3–4 minutes. Serve immediately.

Vegetarian Option

Sweet and Sour Vegetables

Serves 4

½ tsp sesame oil
125g/4oz mushrooms, sliced
1 medium courgette, sliced
1 large carrot, chopped
1 large red pepper, chopped
175g/6oz broccoli florets
125g/4oz bean sprouts

2 cloves garlic, crushed
¼ tsp chilli powder
25g/1oz fresh root ginger, peeled and chopped

Sauce

4 tbsp white wine vinegar
2 tbsp cornflour
2 tbsp soy sauce
25g/1oz brown sugar
2 tbsp tomato purée

1. Heat the sesame oil gently, add the vegetables, garlic, chilli and ginger and cook for several minutes, stirring continually (other vegetables may also be used, such as baby sweetcorn and mangetout). Remove the vegetables in to a separate dish.
2. Make the sauce as described above.
3. Replace the vegetables to the pan with the sauce and cook for 3–4 minutes. Serve immediately.

DAY 2

LUNCH

Vegetable Soup

Serves 4

2 medium potatoes, chopped finely
2 medium carrots, chopped finely
1 onion, chopped finely
1 leek, chopped finely
1 parsnip, chopped finely
1–2 cups water or vegetable stock
1 bay leaf
parsley, to taste
pinch of salt and pepper

1. Take the vegetables and cover with the water or stock. Add the bay leaf, parsley, salt and pepper.
2. Cook slowly (simmer) for 45 minutes, then liquidize until smooth and serve.
   Can be frozen.

DINNER

Smoked Mackerel with Pasta

Serves 4

4 large peppered smoked mackerel fillets
2 tbsp lemon juice
1 tbsp capers, chopped
1 large sprig of basil, shredded
4 tbsp chopped parsley
2 tbsp snipped chives
500g/1lb pasta
150g/5oz low-fat fromage frais
pinch of salt

1. Remove the skin and bones from the mackerel and flake. Mix in the lemon juice, capers and herbs and place in a warm bowl.
2. Meanwhile, cook the pasta as per the instructions and adding the salt, rinse and drain thoroughly.
3. Fold the fromage frais into the pasta and then finally fold in the mackerel. Serve immediately.

DAY 3

LUNCH

Jacket Potato

Select a filling from pages 166–7.

DINNER

Lasagne

Serves 4

125g/4oz fresh or packet lasagne
500g/1lb lean minced beef or turkey

Red Sauce

1 large onion, chopped finely
25g/1oz mushrooms, chopped finely
1 red pepper, chopped finely
2 carrots, chopped finely
2 celery sticks, chopped finely
425g/14oz tinned chopped tomatoes
1 tsp chopped fresh/½ tsp dried marjoram
1 tsp chopped fresh/½ tsp dried basil
1 clove garlic, crushed

1 tsp tomato purée
salt and pepper
300ml/½ pint stock, meat or vegetable

White Sauce

300ml/½ pint skimmed milk
50g/2oz cornflour
salt and pepper
15g/½ oz butter
50g/2oz low-fat cheese, grated

Topping

125g/4oz cottage cheese

1. Preheat the oven to 170ºC/325ºF/gas mark 3.
2. Take the vegetables for the red sauce and sauté
    in a heavy-based pan in 1 tbsp of water. Add the
    tinned tomatoes, herbs, garlic, tomato purée, salt
    and pepper.
3. Add the meat and stock and stir well. Pour the
    sauce into an ovenproof dish and place in the
    oven for 1 hour or until the sauce has thickened.
    Alternatively, cook in a saucepan on top of the
    oven on a low/moderate heat for 20 minutes,
    stirring regularly.
4. When this is nearly ready, prepare the white
    sauce. Place 4 tbsp of the milk into a bowl and
    add the cornflour, salt and pepper to make a

smooth paste. Put the remaining milk and the butter into a pan and heat gently before adding the cheese – do not allow to boil. Pour the warm milk and butter into the cornflour mixture, mix well and return to the pan. Stir until smooth and thick.

5. Place a layer of the red sauce containing the meat into the bottom of an ovenproof dish, cover with lasagne and then red sauce again. Follow this with a layer of white sauce, another layer of lasagne and then cover completely with the cottage cheese. Place in the oven and cook for approximately 30 minutes at 150ºC/300ºF/gas mark 2.

Vegetarian Option

Vegetarian Lasagne

Replace the meat with 500g/1lb mixed vegetables of your choice, such as mushrooms, onions, carrots, peppers (green or red) or courgettes. Prepare as above.

DAY 4

LUNCH

Sandwich

Select a filling from page 166–7.

DINNER

Chicken Curry

Serves 4

1 tsp sunflower oil
3 skinless chicken fillets, cubed
1 large onion, chopped
1 clove garlic, crushed
1 large potato, parboiled in the skin and chopped
425g/14oz tinned chopped tomatoes
2 tbsp mango chutney
salt and pepper
1 tsp curry paste (optional)
2 tbsp mild curry powder
150ml/¼ pint chicken stock
3 lemon slices

1. Preheat the oven to 170°C/325°F/gas mark 3.
2. Heat the oil gently in a pan, add the meat and brown on both sides. Remove from the pan.
3. Add the onion, garlic and potato to the pan and sauté gently for 2–3 minutes, stirring continually. Mix in the tomatoes and chutney and continue to stir. Add salt and pepper to taste.
4. In a separate jug, add the curry paste and powder to the chicken stock and mix well. Pour over the mixture in the pan.
5. Replace the chicken, add the lemon slices, cover and place in the oven for 30–40 minutes.

Vegetarian Option

Vegetable Curry

Replace the chicken fillets with approximately 300g/10oz of root vegetables, such as carrots, swede or parsnips, and the chicken stock with vegetable stock. Prepare as above.

DAY 5

LUNCH

Pasta Salad

Serves 1

25g–50g/1–2oz durum-wheat pasta
1 tbsp fat-free salad dressing
1 apple, chopped
1 small beetroot, chopped
1 celery stick, chopped
½ tsp chopped fresh mint or chives

1. Cook the pasta as per the instructions and drain.
2. Add the dressing to the pasta and stir well.
3. Add the chopped apple, beetroot and celery and garnish with the mint/chives.

DINNER

Cider Fish Bake

Serves 4

250g/8oz leeks, chopped into large chunks
2 carrots, chopped into large chunks

1 clove garlic, crushed
150ml/¼ pint fish or vegetable stock
1 tbsp cornflour
150ml/¼ pint dry cider
500g/1lb whiting or monkfish
25g/1oz low-fat cheese, grated
125g/4oz fresh breadcrumbs
1 tsp sesame seeds
salt and pepper

1. Preheat the oven to 200ºC/400ºF/gas mark 6.
2. Place the leeks and carrots in a heavy-based pan and add the garlic. Add 4 tbsp of the stock, cover and cook for 10 minutes or until leeks are soft.
3. Add the remaining stock. Blend the cornflour with the cider, remove 2 tbsp of hot vegetable stock and add to the cider mixture. Pour the cider mixture onto the vegetables and bring to the boil gently
4. Cube the fish and place in an ovenproof dish. Cover with the vegetable mixture.
5. Mix the remaining ingredients together, adding salt and pepper to taste, and sprinkle over the top. Bake for 25–30 minutes or until golden brown.

DAY 6

LUNCH

Stuffed Tomato

Serves 1

50g/2oz button mushrooms, chopped
25g/1oz breadcrumbs
zest of ½ lemon
1 tbsp lemon juice
salt and black pepper
1 dstsp fromage frais or cottage cheese
1 large beefsteak tomato

1. Preheat the oven to 140ºC/275ºF/gas mark 1.
2. Grill the mushrooms and add to the breadcrumbs.
3. Add the zest and juice of the lemon. Season well with plenty of black pepper and salt to taste and mix everything together with the fromage frais/cheese.
4. Scoop out most of the tomato flesh, replace with the filling and bake for 20 minutes.

DINNER

Spaghetti Bolognese

Serves 4

450g/15oz spaghetti or tagliatelle
500g/1lb lean minced beef or turkey

Red Sauce

1 large onion, chopped finely
25g/1oz mushrooms, chopped finely
1 red pepper, chopped finely
2 carrots, chopped finely
2 celery sticks, chopped finely
425g/14oz tinned chopped tomatoes
½ tsp marjoram
1 tsp chopped fresh/½ tsp dried basil
1 clove garlic, crushed
1 tsp tomato purée
salt and pepper
300ml/½ pint stock, meat or vegetable

1. Prepare the red sauce as on page 186.
2. Cook the pasta, rinse and drain well.
3. Place the pasta in a bowl and top with the red
   sauce. Serve immediately.

DAY 7

LUNCH

Waldorf Salad

Serves 1

1 medium red apple, cored and diced
1 tbsp lemon juice, fresh or bottled
50g/2oz celery, diced
2 tbsp low-fat yogurt or fat-free fromage frais
crisp lettuce leaves
4 walnut halves, crushed

1. Toss the diced apple in lemon juice to prevent discoloration. Drain well and then mix with the celery.
2. Add the yogurt/fromage frais and toss through the salad, ensuring that all the ingredients are coated with the mixture.
3. Arrange salad on a bed of crisp lettuce leaves and sprinkle with walnuts just before serving.

DINNER

Italian Chicken Casserole

Serves 4

2 tsp extra virgin olive oil
4 chicken portions
1 clove garlic, crushed
1 medium onion, chopped
125g/4oz mushrooms, sliced
425g/14oz tinned chopped tomatoes
½ small green pepper, sliced
½ red pepper, chopped
1 tbsp chopped fresh parsley, plus a little extra for
    sprinkling
½ tsp dried thyme
3 tbsp red wine
salt and pepper

1. Preheat the oven to 180ºC/350ºF/gas mark 4.
2. Heat the oil gently in a large frying pan and then brown the chicken pieces. Transfer them to an ovenproof casserole dish.
3. Add the garlic, onion and mushrooms to the juices in the pan and sauté gently until tender. Add all the remaining ingredients and bring to the boil, stirring continually.

4. Pour the sauce over the chicken, cover and cook in the oven for 60 minutes. Garnish with the extra chopped parsley.

Vegetarian Option

Vegetable Casserole

Replace the chicken with 175–250g/6–8oz of vegetables, such as aubergines and courgettes, and add 425g/14oz tinned, drained borlotti beans. Prepare as above.

DAY 8

LUNCH

Mini Pizza with Mushrooms and Peppers

Serves 1

15cm/6in pizza base
4 button mushrooms, chopped
½ pepper, chopped
½–1 level tbsp low-fat cheese, grated

1. Cover the pizza base with the toppings.
2. Grill or bake according to the instructions on the pizza packet.

DINNER

Spicy Fish Dish

Serves 4

1 tsp olive oil
1 small onion, chopped finely
2 cloves garlic, crushed
1 tbsp fresh root ginger, chopped finely
4 green cardamom pods
1 tsp ground turmeric
1 tsp ground cumin
2 tbsp ground coriander
150ml/¼ pint plain yogurt
salt and pepper
4 whiting fillets, skinned

1. Preheat the oven to 180ºC/350ºF/gas mark 4.
2. Place the oil in a heavy-based pan and add the onion, garlic and ginger. Cook gently for 2–3 minutes, stirring continuously.
3. Remove the pan from the heat. Place the cardamom pods in the mixture, add the turmeric, cumin and coriander and cook for 2–3 minutes, stirring well.
4. Allow the mixture to cool, then stir in the yogurt and seasoning.

5. Place the fish fillets in to a large, shallow, ovenproof dish and spread the spicy mixture evenly over each fillet. Cover and cook for 10 minutes.

DAY 9

LUNCH

Jacket Potato

Select a filling from pages 166–7.

DINNER

Chicken and Pineapple

Serves 4

2 tsp olive oil
4 skinless chicken fillets
1 onion, chopped
1 tsp chopped fresh/½ tsp dried thyme
1 large clove garlic, crushed
½ tsp ground ginger
¼ tsp ground cinnamon
pinch of ground cloves

425g/14oz tinned pineapple slices in natural juice,
  drained
200g/7oz tinned tomatoes
90ml/3fl oz red wine
salt and pepper

1. Preheat the oven to 170ºC/325ºF/gas mark 3.
2. Heat the oil and fry the chicken gently on both
   sides for 3 minutes, stirring to avoid sticking.
   Transfer to another dish.
3. Now add the onion and thyme to the pan and
   sauté gently until soft. Add the garlic, ginger,
   cinnamon and cloves and cook for 2–3 minutes.
4. Chop the pineapple and mix with the tinned
   tomatoes, wine and seasoning. Add to the
   mixture in the pan and cook gently for
   2–3 minutes.
5. Place some of the mixture in an ovenproof dish,
   slice the chicken and place on top, followed by
   the remaining mixture. Cover and bake for
   approximately 40 minutes.

Vegetarian Option

Chick Pea and Mushroom Curry

Serves 4

2 tsp olive oil
250g/8oz button mushrooms, quartered

1 small onion, chopped

2 cloves garlic, chopped

1 small piece fresh root ginger, peeled and chopped

425g/14 oz tinned chick peas, drained

400g/13oz tinned tomatoes

1 tsp ground coriander

40g/1½ oz cashew nuts

125ml/4fl oz vegetable stock

1 tsp mild curry paste

2 tsp hot or medium curry powder

4 tbsp Greek yogurt

2 tbsp chopped fresh coriander (optional)

1. Heat the oil gently in a pan and sauté the mushrooms, onion, garlic and ginger for 2–3 minutes.
2. Add the chick peas, tomatoes, ground coriander and cashew nuts to the mixture.
3. In a jug, put the stock, curry paste and curry powder. Mix well and pour over the chick pea mixture. Cook gently for 6–8 minutes or until the mixture has thickened.
4. Remove from the heat and stir in the yogurt and fresh coriander. Return to a gentle heat for 2–3 minutes (do not allow to boil) and serve.

DAY 10

LUNCH

Stir-Fried Vegetables in Pitta Bread

Serves 1

½ carrot, chopped
⅓ cucumber, sliced lengthways
25g/1oz spring onions, chopped
4 whole baby sweetcorn
15g/½oz beansprouts
generous dash soy sauce
1 pitta bread

1. Cook the vegetables gently in 1 tbsp of water and soy sauce for 3–4 minutes.
2. Place the mixture in the pitta bread and serve.

DINNER

Piquant Pork

Serves 4

1 tsp olive oil
4 tender pork steaks (all fat removed)
1 large onion, chopped

1 clove garlic, crushed
1 tbsp plain or self-raising flour
1 tsp hot paprika
425g/14oz tinned chopped tomatoes
1 tbsp tomato purée
½ tbsp brown sugar
2 tbsp wine vinegar
salt and pepper

1. Preheat the oven to 180ºC/350ºF/gas mark 4.
2. Heat the oil gently in a large pan and brown the pork steaks on both sides. Transfer to a large, ovenproof casserole dish.
3. Add the onion and garlic to the pan and sauté for 3 minutes.
4. Remove the pan from the heat, add the flour and paprika and mix well. Return to the heat and continue to stir for 1 minute.
5. Add the tomatoes, purée, sugar, wine vinegar and salt and pepper to taste. Stir well as you bring to the boil. Pour over the pork steaks, cover and cook for 1 hour.

Vegetarian Option

Vegetables in Piquant Sauce

Serves 4

Replace the pork with 150g/5oz cauliflower florets

and 150g/5oz broccoli florets. Prepare the sauce as above and place the cauliflower and broccoli in an ovenproof dish. Stir 25g/1oz whole almonds into the sauce and pour over the broccoli and cauliflower. Cover and cook for 30 minutes.

DAY 11

LUNCH

Sandwich

Select a filling from pages 166–7.

DINNER

Stir-Fried Beef, Chicken or Turkey in Black Bean Sauce

1 tsp sesame oil
375g/12oz beef, chicken or turkey, sliced very thinly
3 spring onions, chopped
½ red pepper, sliced
1 carrot, sliced thinly
½ celery stick, sliced thinly
50g/2oz mushrooms, sliced thinly
1 small onion, sliced

1 clove garlic
1 tsp ground ginger
2 tbsp soy sauce
1 tsp cornflour
1 tbsp sherry
1–2 tbsp black bean sauce
1 cup meat or vegetable stock

1. Heat the oil gently and stir-fry the meat for
   2–3 minutes, stirring continuously. Remove from
   the pan.
2. Now sauté all the vegetables gently for 2–3
   minutes, remove and place with the meat.
3. Add the garlic, ginger and soy sauce to the pan
   and cook for 1–2 minutes, stirring constantly.
4. In a separate bowl, put the cornflour and sherry
   and mix to a smooth paste. Stir in the black bean
   sauce.
5. Add the stock to the ginger and garlic in the pan
   and bring to the boil. Take 2 tbsp of this hot
   liquid and add to the cornflour mixture. Pour
   this cornflour mixture into the pan and stir until
   thickened. Return the meat and vegetables to the
   pan and heat thoroughly.

Vegetarian Option

Stir-Fried Vegetables in Black Bean Sauce

Replace the meat with 500g/1lb of vegetables, such as beansprouts, mangetout, carrots, cucumber, spring onions, celery, baby sweetcorn and red pepper. Prepare as above, but when stir-frying your chosen vegetables, add 125g/4oz chick peas to the mixture.

DAY 12

LUNCH

Beans on Toast

2 thick slices of toast (without butter) with a small tin of baked beans.

DINNER

Fish Plaki

Serves 4

750g/1½lb fresh or frozen trout, cod or haddock, skinned

1 tbsp olive oil
1 large onion, sliced thinly
1 clove garlic, crushed
4 tbsp chopped fresh parsley,
425g/14oz tinned, chopped tomatoes
1 tbsp lemon juice
salt and pepper
4 lemon slices

1. Preheat the oven to 180ºC/350ºF/gas mark 4.
2. Cut the fish into four portions and place in a large, shallow ovenproof dish.
3. Heat the oil gently before adding the onion, garlic and parsley. Sauté for 2–3 minutes. Add the tomatoes, lemon juice and seasoning and bring to the boil.
4. Pour over the fish and place the lemon slices ontop. Cover and cook in the oven for 25 minutes. Remove the cover and cook for a further 10–15 minutes.

DAY 13

LUNCH

Sandwich

Select a filling from pages 166–7.

DINNER

Chilli Con Carne

Serves 4

1 tbsp olive oil
1 clove garlic, crushed
1 medium onion, chopped
125g/4oz mushrooms, chopped
1 red pepper, sliced
425g/14oz tinned chopped tomatoes
500g/1lb lean minced beef
1–2 tbsp tomato purée
450g/15oz tinned red kidney beans
1 tbsp chilli powder
1 tsp chilli sauce
salt and pepper

1. Heat the oil gently in a pan and add the garlic.
   Sauté the onion, mushrooms and pepper for
   2–3 minutes, stirring continuously. Add the
   tinned tomatoes and cook for a further minute.
   Remove and place in a bowl.
2. Fry the meat gently in the vegetable juices for
   3–4 minutes, stirring continually. Replace the
   vegetables and mix in with the meat, before
   adding the purée and the kidney beans.

3. Mix the chilli powder and chilli sauce together in a separate cup, then stir into the mixture, adding salt and pepper to taste. Cover and cook for 30 minutes on a very low heat.

Vegetarian Option

Vegetarian Chilli

Replace the mince with 500g/1lb of vegetables, such as mashed swede, grated carrot and aubergine. Prepare as above.

DAY 14

LUNCH

Curried Parsnip Soup

Serves 4

3 parsnips, chopped
1 large onion, chopped
1 tbsp curry powder/sauce
150ml/¼ pint milk
150ml/¼ pint water
chopped fresh coriander (optional), to taste

1. Place the parsnips and onion in a heavy-based

pan with the curry powder/sauce, stir well and
cook for 2–3 minutes in a tbsp of water.

2. Add the milk and water and cook on a low heat
for a further 45 minutes. Liquidize and serve.
The coriander can be added for extra flavour.
Can be frozen.

DINNER

Autumn Pie

Serves 4

1 tsp olive oil
1 large onion, chopped
2 large carrots, cut into thick sticks
125g/4oz courgettes, cut into thick sticks
400g/13oz tinned chopped tomatoes
300g/10oz lean minced beef, dry-fried in a non-stick
    pan and drained of fat
salt and pepper
3 tbsp frozen peas
375g/12oz potatoes, peeled
3 tbsp fresh breadcrumbs

1. Preheat the oven to 170ºC/325ºF/gas mark 3.
2. Heat the oil gently and sauté the onion for
2–3 minutes. Add the carrots, courgettes and
tomatoes and cook for a further 2–3 minutes.

Remove from the pan and place in a bowl.

3. Sauté the mince gently until browned, stirring all the time. Replace the vegetables and continue to cook. Season to taste, add the peas and leave on a low heat for 10 minutes.

4. Meanwhile, boil and mash the potatoes. Place the meat in an ovenproof dish, spread the potato on top and sprinkle with the breadcrumbs. Cook in the oven for 50–60 minutes.

Vegetarian Option

Leek and Bean Macaroni

Serves 4

375g/12oz wholewheat macaroni
1 tsp olive oil
375g/12oz leeks, sliced thinly
425g/14oz tinned mixed beans
1 tsp coarse-grain mustard
125g/4oz cottage cheese

White Sauce

300ml/½ pint skimmed milk
50g/2oz cornflour
salt and pepper
15g/½oz butter
50g/2oz low-fat cheese, grated

1. Preheat the oven to 220°C/425°F/gas mark 7.
2. Cook the macaroni as per the instructions on the packet, rinse and drain.
3. Heat the oil in a heavy-based pan and sauté the leeks for 3–4 minutes.
4. Remove the pan from the heat and add the beans, leaving 1 tbsp of the bean water to mix together with the mustard. Add this to the leek/bean mixture.
5. Prepare the white sauce as on page 186. Mix the macaroni in with the white sauce and add this to the bean mixture. Stir well and remove from the pan and place in a large ovenproof dish. Top with the cottage cheese and bake for 20 minutes.

DAY 15

LUNCH

Sandwich

Select a filling from page 166–7.

DINNER

Chilli Chicken with Orange

Serves 4

2 onions, sliced
1 red pepper, sliced
125g/4oz mushrooms, sliced
425g/14oz tinned chilli beans
400g/13oz tinned tomatoes
salt and pepper
2 tsp tomato purée
1 sprig of parsley, chopped
½ tsp chilli powder
4 chicken fillets
2 oranges

1. Place the onions, pepper and mushrooms in a casserole pan with a thick bottom. Sweat the vegetables for 5 minutes, stirring all the time.
2. Add the chilli beans, tomatoes, salt, pepper, tomato purée, parsley and chilli powder.
3. Grill the chicken pieces for about 2 minutes, to just seal the outside.
4. Squeeze the juice from 1 orange into the vegetable mixture and then add the chicken pieces. Top with a layer of sliced orange from

the remaining orange. Cover the casserole and
cook for 1½–2 hours over a low heat or until
the sauce is thick. Serve with rice.

Vegetarian Option

Vegetables in Chilli and Orange Sauce

Replace the chicken with 500g/1lb of root vegetables,
such as swede and carrots. Prepare as above, but add
125g/4oz of cooked lentils 10 minutes before serving.

DAY 16

LUNCH

Vegetable and Bean Soup

Serves 4

1 tbsp olive oil
1 large onion, chopped roughly
1 large parsnip, peeled and chopped roughly
1 large carrot, peeled and chopped roughly
1 large potato, peeled and chopped roughly
2 courgettes, sliced thinly
300–600ml/½–1 pint vegetable stock
1–2 tsp mild curry paste
1 clove garlic, crushed

450g/15oz tinned red kidney beans, drained and
 rinsed
450g/15 oz tinned black-eyed beans, drained and
 rinsed
salt and pepper
3 tbsp chopped fresh coriander

1. Heat the oil gently and sauté the vegetables for
 3–4 minutes.
2. In a separate bowl, mix together the stock, curry
 paste and garlic and pour this onto the
 vegetables. Stir and simmer for 25–30 minutes or
 until the vegetables are tender. (You can purée
 the mixture at this stage if a smoother texture is
 preferred.)
3. Mix in the beans and season to taste, before
 adding the coriander. Simmer for 10 minutes
 and serve.

DINNER

Tuna Salad

Serves 4

375g/12oz spinach pasta shapes
25g/1oz pine nuts/almonds

250g/½lb tomatoes, chopped into wedges
425g/14oz tinned tuna in spring water
4 tbsp chopped fresh basil
Italian garlic dressing (fat free)

1. Cook the pasta as per the instructions, rinse and drain.
2. Brown the nuts on a baking tray in the oven. Drain the tuna and mix everything together with the dressing. Serve immediately.

DAY 17

LUNCH

Tasty Tomatoes on Toast

Serves 1

1 slice thickly cut bread
200g/7oz tinned tomatoes
pinch of fresh basil
25g/1oz low-fat cottage cheese

1. Brown the bread on one side and mix the tomatoes and basil together before spreading on the other side.

2. Place the cottage cheese on top of the tomatoes and grill for 2–3 minutes.

DINNER

Shepherd's Pie

Serves 4

375–500g/12oz–1lb lean minced beef
750g/1½lb potatoes

Red Sauce

1 large onion, chopped finely
25g/1oz mushrooms, chopped finely
1 red pepper, chopped finely
2 carrots, chopped finely
2 celery sticks, chopped finely
425g/14oz tinned chopped tomatoes
½ tsp marjoram
1 tsp chopped fresh/½ tsp dried basil
1 clove garlic, crushed
1 tsp tomato purée
salt and pepper
300ml/½ pint stock, meat or vegetable

1. Preheat the oven to 220ºC/425ºF/gas mark 7
2. Prepare the red sauce as on page 186 and pour

the cooked red sauce containing the meat into a deep ovenproof dish.

3. Cook and mash the potatoes and cover the red sauce with them. Place in the oven for 30 minutes or until the potato browns.

Vegetarian Option

Vegetarian Shepherd's Pie

Serves 4

Replace the meat with approximately 750g/1½lb tinned mixed, cannelloni or kidney beans. Prepare as above.

DAY 18

LUNCH

Mini Pizza with Sweetcorn and Green Beans

Serves 1

15cm/6in pizza base
1–2 dstsp sweetcorn
1–2 dstsp tinned green beans

Prepare as on page 196. If you wish, top with ½–1 level tsp of low-fat cottage cheese.

DINNER

Beef Stew with Cider

Serves 4

500g/1lb rump steak, cut into cubes
1 large onion, chopped roughly
2 carrots, chopped roughly
2 turnips, chopped roughly
2 celery sticks, chopped roughly
600ml/1 pint stock, meat or vegetable
1 tbsp flour, seasoned with salt and pepper
150ml/¼ pint cider

1. Preheat the oven to 150ºC/300ºF/gas mark 2.
2. Place the meat and vegetables in a pan and add 4 tbsp of the stock. Cook for 5–6 minutes and remove from the heat.
3. In a separate bowl, put the flour and 2 tbsp of stock and mix to a paste. Pour the remaining stock over the meat and vegetables, stirring well.
4. Pour the flour mixture back into the pan with the meat and vegetables. Stir well and cook until the sauce thickens. Add the cider and put the mixture into an ovenproof dish, cover and cook for 1–1½ hours.

Vegetarian Option

Vegetable and Nut Stir-Fry

Serves 4

1 tsp sesame oil
125g/4oz baby sweetcorn
1 large red pepper, seeded and cut into strips
150g/5oz mangetout
1 bunch spring onions, shredded
300g/10oz button mushrooms, sliced
25g/1oz fresh root ginger, grated
4 tbsp soy sauce
½ tbsp set honey
1 tbsp cornflour
1 tbsp tomato purée
1 cup vegetable stock
250g/8oz bean sprouts
50g/2oz split cashew nuts

1. Heat the oil in a wok or large frying pan. Add
   the corn, pepper and mangetout. Then add the
   onions, mushrooms and ginger and stir-fry for
   2–3 minutes. Remove the vegetables from the
   pan and place in a bowl.
2. Put the soy sauce and honey into the pan.
3. In a separate bowl, put the cornflour, tomato
   purée and 1 tbsp of the vegetable stock. Mix

these to a smooth paste.

4. Heat the soy sauce and the honey and pour onto the cornflour mixture, then pour this mixture back into the pan and cook to a smooth paste.

5. Stir in the beansprouts and cook for 2 minutes. Add the vegetables and nuts and cook for a further 5 minutes. Serve immediately.

DAY 19

LUNCH

Jacket Potato

Select a filling from page 166–7.

DINNER

Crunchy Fish Dish

Serves 4

50g/2oz fresh breadcrumbs
1 tsp mustard powder
4 tbsp bran flakes or cornflakes, crushed
1 tbsp low-fat cheese, grated
1 tbsp chopped fresh parsley

1 tsp dried thyme
zest of 1 lemon
1 tsp olive oil and a little lemon juice, mixed together
750g/1½lb cod fillet, skinned and cut into four pieces
salt and pepper

1. Preheat the oven to 180ºC/350ºF/gas mark 4.
2. Mix together the breadcrumbs, mustard, bran flakes or cornflakes, low-fat cheese, parsley, thyme and lemon zest.
3. Brush an ovenproof dish with the olive oil and lemon juice before laying the pieces of fish in it. Brush the fish with the same mixture and sprinkle with seasoning.
4. Coat each piece of fish with the breadcrumb mixture, cover and bake for 30 minutes or until the topping is brown and the fish cooked.

DAY 20

LUNCH

Tomato and Rice Soup

Serves 4

1 large onion, chopped finely
1 large carrot, chopped finely

425g/14oz tinned chopped tomatoes
1 tsp olive oil
900ml/1½ pint chicken or vegetable stock
¼ tsp dried marjoram
salt and pepper
2 tbsp uncooked wholegrain rice
1 tbsp chopped fresh parsley

1. Place the onion, carrot and tomatoes into a pan
    with the olive oil and sauté gently for 5 minutes.
2. Add all the remaining ingredients, except the rice
    and parsley, and bring to the boil. Cover and
    simmer for 30 minutes.
3. Add the rice and simmer for a further
    12 minutes. Stir in the parsley just before serving.
    Can be frozen.

DINNER

Chicken in Barbecue Sauce

Serves 4

1 tsp olive oil
1 large onion, chopped
4 skinned chicken fillets
425g/14oz tinned chopped tomatoes
1 tsp English mustard
1 tbsp brown sugar

2 tbsp wine vinegar
2 tbsp Worcestershire sauce
¼ tsp garlic powder
¼ tsp salt
1 tsp chilli powder
2 tsp tomato purée

1. Heat the oil and sauté the onion until golden brown. Add the chicken fillets and fry gently for approximately 5 minutes or until browned.
2. Add all the remaining ingredients and bring to the boil, stirring continuously. Cover and simmer for 25 minutes.
3. Either serve as it is or purée for a smoother sauce. Serve with the chicken. (The barbecue sauce can also be used as a topping for jacket potatoes.)

Vegetarian Option

Courgette and Carrot Loaf

Serves 4

1 small onion
25g/1oz nuts (almonds or other)
125g/4oz courgettes, trimmed and grated
125g/4oz carrots, grated
25g/1oz porridge oats

1 tbsp tomato purée
¼ tsp dried mixed herbs
salt and black pepper

1. Preheat the oven to 180ºC/350ºF/gas mark 4.
2. Sauté the onion gently for 5 minutes. Add the nuts, courgettes and carrots and cook for 5 minutes.
3. Stir in the remaining ingredients and spoon the mixture into a non-stick 1kg/2lb-loaf tin, pressing down well.
4. Cook near the top of the oven for approximately 25 minutes or until brown. Allow to cool for 3–5 minutes before turning out and serving.

DAY 21

LUNCH

Sandwich

Select a filling from page 166–7.

DINNER

Sweet Pork or Chicken Pot

Serves 4

1 tsp olive oil
500g/1lb pork fillet or chicken, cubed
1 red pepper, sliced
1 green pepper, sliced
1 onion, chopped
25g/1oz potatoes, sliced
1 tbsp tomato purée
50 ml/¼ pint white wine
3 tbsp pineapple juice
sprig of fresh thyme
salt and pepper
300ml/½ pint chicken stock
2 tbsp cornflour
125g/4oz sweetcorn
125g/4oz pineapple, diced
1 tbsp chopped fresh parsley

1. Heat the oil gently and sauté the meat, peppers
   onion and potatoes. Stir continually and cook for
   5–6 minutes.
2. Add the tomato purée, white wine, pineapple
   juice, thyme, salt and pepper and bring to the boil.

3. Use 4 tbsp of the stock with the cornflour to make a smooth paste and add the remaining stock to the vegetables and meat.
4. Heat the meat and vegetable mixture gently for 20 minutes. Stir in the cornflour mixture and simmer for 3 minutes or until the sauce has thickened.
5. Add the sweetcorn, pineapple and parsley, and stir and simmer for 3 minutes.

Vegetarian Option

Spicy Peas and Potatoes

Serves 4

1 tsp olive oil
2 large onions, chopped
1 clove garlic, crushed
6 green cardamom pods
2 tbsp cumin seeds
25g/1oz fresh root ginger, peeled and chopped
1 green chilli, seeded and chopped
1 bay leaf
1kg/2lb potatoes, cubed
1 tsp turmeric
salt and pepper
150ml/¼ pint vegetable stock
375g/12oz frozen peas
150ml/¼ pint plain yogurt

50g/2oz chopped nuts (preferably almonds)

1. Heat the oil gently in a saucepan. Add the onions, garlic, cardamom pods, cumin, ginger, chilli and bay leaf to the pan and sauté for 10 minutes, stirring continuously.
2. Add the potatoes, turmeric and seasoning, and pour in the stock. Cover and simmer for 15 minutes.
3. Stir in the peas and simmer for a further 10–15 minutes or until the potatoes are soft.
4. Add the yogurt while still heating gently (do not boil). Sprinkle with the chopped nuts just before serving.

DAY 22

LUNCH

Tomato Soup

Serves 4–6

1 tsp olive oil
1 medium onion, chopped
1 medium carrot, chopped
1 celery stick, chopped
425g/14oz tinned chopped tomatoes

900ml/1½ pint chicken or vegetable stock
1 medium potato, chopped
2 tsp tomato purée
pinch of
salt and pepper
150ml/¼ pint long-life skimmed milk

1. Heat the oil gently in a large pan, add the vegetables and sauté for 10 minutes.
2. Add the tomatoes, stock, potato, purée, tarragon and seasoning. Cover and simmer for 45 minutes.
3. Pureé the mixture, stir in the milk and reheat to serve.
   Can be frozen.

DINNER

Moussaka

Serves 4

2 medium aubergines, sliced
salt
2 medium onions, sliced
500g/1lb minced beef
400g/13oz tinned tomatoes
1 tbsp chopped parsley
pinch of nutmeg

1 clove garlic
pepper
2 tbsp tomato purée
300ml/½ pint low-fat yogurt
1 tbsp cottage cheese

1. Sprinkle the aubergines with salt and leave for 30 minutes. Preheat the oven to 150°C/300°F/gas mark 2.
2. Dry sauté the slices of aubergines for 5 minutes and then remove from the pan.
3. Sauté the onions and beef and add the tomatoes, parsley, nutmeg, garlic, salt, pepper and tomato purée. Simmer for 30 minutes.
4. In an ovenproof dish, place alternate layers of aubergines and meat sauce until the top layer is aubergines.
5. Mix the yogurt and cottage cheese together and pour over the aubergines. Bake for 20 minutes and grill just before serving to brown. Serve with Granary bread and salad.

Vegetarian Option

Vegetarian Moussaka

Prepare as above, but replace the beef with 500g/1lb root vegetables, cooked and mashed.

DAY 23

LUNCH

Jacket Potato

Select a filling from page 166–7.

DINNER

Smoked Haddock Loaf

Serves 4

750g/1½lb smoked haddock or cod
150ml/¼ pint milk
salt and pepper
2 eggs
50g/2oz low-fat Cheddar cheese, grated
1 sprig of parsley, chopped

White Sauce

25g/1oz cornflour
25g/1oz butter

1. Preheat the oven to 150ºC/300ºF/gas mark 2.
2. Place the fish in a dish with the milk and salt and

pepper to taste and cook for approximately
20 minutes until tender. Separate the eggs and
add the flaked fish to the egg yolks.

3. Prepare the white sauce as on page 186, but
using the milk from the cooked fish. Add the
cheese, parsley and the fish mixture.

4. Whisk the egg whites until very stiff and fold
into the fish mixture. Place in a 1kg/2lb-loaf
tin lined with foil (or a mould), and bake for 30
minutes.

5. Turn out onto a plate and slice.

DAY 24

LUNCH

Vegetable Rice

Serves 1

250g/8oz frozen rice with peas and mushrooms
Carrots, sliced and sweetcorn, as desired

1. Sauté everything gently with water (not oil as
directed on some rice packets) until soft.

2. Serve immediately.

DINNER

Steamed Ginger Chicken

Serves 4

4 chicken fillets, skinned
4 tbsp sherry
3 tbsp soy sauce
8 spring onions, cut into small slices
50g/2oz fresh root ginger, peeled and chopped

1. Place the chicken in an ovenproof dish.
2. Mix the sherry and soy sauce together and add the onions and ginger.
3. Spoon the mixture over the chicken, cover and marinate for several hours (or overnight) in the fridge.
4. Turn the chicken fillets over and cover the dish with foil. Cook at 150ºC/300ºF/gas mark 2 for 45 minutes or until the chicken is tender.

Vegetarian Option

Stuffed Mushrooms

Serves 4

1 tsp olive oil
1 clove garlic, crushed

1 small onion, very finely chopped
75g/3oz fresh breadcrumbs
2 pineapple rings, chopped
250g/8oz cottage cheese
salt and pepper
grated nutmeg
8 large, flat mushrooms, stalks removed

1. Preheat the oven to 200ºC/400ºF/gas mark 6.
2. Heat the oil gently in a pan and add the garlic and onion. Stir-fry until the onion is soft and then add the breadcrumbs.
3. Stir in the pineapple and cottage cheese, salt, pepper and nutmeg to taste.
4. Place the mushrooms in an ovenproof dish and fill each one with the stuffing. Bake for 20–25 minutes.

DAY 25

LUNCH

Pizza Bread and Tuna

Serves 1

Prepare as on page 179, but adding 25g/1oz of tuna.

DINNER

Fruity Chicken Biryani

Serves 4

1 tsp olive oil
25g/1oz onion, finely chopped
1 clove garlic, crushed
1 red pepper, seeded and chopped
200ml/7fl oz chicken stock
½ tsp turmeric
1 tbsp curry paste
300g/10oz boned chicken, skin removed and
   cubed
50g/2oz apricots
25g/1oz raisins
75g/3oz long-grain rice
2 tsp low-sugar apricot jam
pinch of salt and pepper
1 tbsp flaked almonds
6 tbsp low-fat yogurt
2 tbsp finely chopped cucumber

1. Heat the oil gently and add the onion, garlic and
   red pepper and cook for 2–3 minutes.
2. In a separate bowl, mix the chicken stock, turmeric
   and curry paste. Pour over the onion mixture.

3. Add the chicken, simmer for 8–10 minutes and then add the apricots, raisins, rice, jam and salt and pepper to taste. Bring to the boil, stir and cover. Simmer and cook for 20 minutes or until the rice and chicken are tender.

4. Transfer to a serving dish and top with the flaked almonds. Mix the yogurt and cucumber together to add on the side.

Vegetarian Option

Vegetable Biryani

Replace the chicken with 500g/1lb fruity root vegetables, such as parsnips, swede, squash or pumpkin, and the chicken stock with vegetable stock. Prepare as above.

DAY 26

LUNCH

Sandwich

Select a filling from page 166–7.

DINNER

Kedgeree

Serves 4

250g/8oz long-grain brown rice
1 egg
300g/10oz smoked haddock
1 tbsp chopped fresh parsley
juice of ½ lemon
salt and black pepper
15g/½oz butter or 50g/2oz fromage frais

1. Cook the rice as usual, drain and rinse.
2. Hard-boil the egg, chop it into pieces and add with the haddock, parsley and lemon to the rice.
3. When ready to serve, add the butter/fromage frais. Reheat in the microwave or oven and stir well.

DAY 27

LUNCH

Jacket Potato

Select a filling from page 166–7.

DINNER

Lemon Chicken

Serves 4

4 chicken fillets, skinned and cut into strips
1 tsp sesame oil
1 dried red chilli or ¼ tsp chilli powder
1 tsp fresh ginger
1 red pepper, sliced
50g/2oz mushrooms, sliced
5 spring onions, chopped
½ tsp finely chopped garlic
1 tsp cornflour, blended with 1 tsp water
2 tsp dry sherry or rice wine
2 tsp light soy sauce
1–2 tbsp fresh lemon juice
2 tsp brown sugar
zest of 1 lemon
90ml/3fl oz chicken stock or water

1. Sauté the chicken gently in the sesame oil and garlic for 2–3 minutes. Remove from the pan.
2. Add the vegetables, chilli and ginger to the pan and sauté for 2–3 minutes. Remove from the pan.
3. In a separate bowl, put the cornflour and the sherry/rice wine and mix to make a paste.

4. Put the soy sauce, lemon juice, sugar and lemon zest in the pan, simmer for 1 minute, then pour onto the cornflour mixture. Stir well and then return to the pan to make a thick sauce. Add the chicken stock/water.

5. Return the chicken to the pan and cook for 5 minutes. Add the vegetables and cook for a further 5 minutes.

Vegetarian Option

Lentil and Courgette Bake

Serves 4

1 tsp olive oil
1 onion, chopped finely
1 clove garlic, crushed
1 bay leaf
2 celery sticks, sliced thinly
2 carrots, diced
250g/8oz red lentils
600ml/1 pint vegetable stock
500g/1lb courgettes, sliced
salt and pepper
25g/1oz Cheddar cheese, grated
25g/1oz fresh breadcrumbs
pinch of cayenne pepper

1. Heat the oil gently and add the onion, garlic,

bay leaf, celery and carrots. Sauté for 2–3 minutes, add the lentils and stock and bring to the boil.

2. Stir, cover and simmer for 20–25 minutes or until the lentils are soft.
3. Set the oven to 180ºC/350ºF/gas mark 4.
4. Lay half of the courgettes in an ovenproof dish, cover with the lentil mixture, top with the remaining courgettes and sprinkle with seasoning.
5. Mix the cheese, breadcrumbs and cayenne pepper together and spread over the courgettes. Bake for 30–35 minutes.

DAY 28

LUNCH

Sandwich

Select a filling from page 166–7.

DINNER

Meat Loaf

Serves 4

5 slices bread, grated into crumbs
375g/¾lb minced beef
2 tsp tomato purée
1 stock cube
3 carrots, grated
1 small onion, chopped finely
½ red pepper, chopped finely
1 sprig of parsley, chopped
salt and pepper
1 egg

1. Preheat the oven to 180ºC/350ºF/gas mark 4 and line a 500g/1lb-loaf tin with foil.
2. Put all the ingredients into a bowl and mix together with the egg.
3. Place the mixture in the loaf tin and bake for 30 minutes.

Vegetable Casserole

Serves 4–6

2 tsp olive oil
400g/13oz onions, chopped
2 cloves garlic, crushed
2 green peppers, sliced
400g/13oz courgettes, chopped
2 medium aubergines, chopped
200g/7oz mushrooms, sliced
425g/14oz tinned tomatoes
75g/3oz tomato purée
2 bay leaves
1 tbsp chopped fresh parsley
1 tsp chopped fresh marjoram
1 tsp chopped fresh thyme
salt and pepper
300ml/½ pint vegetable stock or water
400g/13oz potatoes, peeled and sliced thinly

1. Preheat the oven to 180°C/350°F/gas mark 4.
2. Heat the oil in the pan and add the onions, garlic, peppers, courgettes, aubergines and mushrooms. Sauté gently for 5 minutes.
3. Now add the tomatoes, purée, herbs and seasoning. Mix well and pour in the stock.
4. Arrange the potatoes on the top and cover and

bake for 1hour. Remove the lid and bake for a further 30 minutes.

AFTER 28 DAYS – WHAT HAPPENS NOW?

As you have read through this book you have learnt a lot about how your body works and what it needs to function properly. You have also learnt about what it doesn't need to function – and that some foods can be quite harmful to your body, as well as making you gain weight.

If you have followed this plan for 28 days, you could simply start again! After all, the recipes are so delicious you could carry on cooking these meals for ever. I hope that you have also learnt enough to be able to adapt some of your own favourite recipes which were not included in the book. Remember, a diet isn't something you 'go on' and then 'come off'. If you have made the important decision to watch what you eat, it doesn't stop here, in fact this is just the beginning.

If you have followed the recipes and done the exercises then you will be feeling fitter by now, you will have more energy, feel less lethargic and generally healthier. Perhaps people are starting to comment on how well you look – you will certainly feel much better. All the good work you have achieved over the past month must be carried on until it becomes a way of life – not a hardship, but a way of living life to the full. If you look after your body it adds years to your life and life to your years! *Go for it*.

INDEX